FEAST
WITHOUT
YEAST

4 STAGES TO BETTER HEALTH

A complete guide to implementing yeast free,
wheat (gluten) free and milk (casein) free living.
Featuring more than **225 original** recipes.

by **BRUCE SEMON, M.D., Ph.D.**
and **LORI KORNBLUM**

Foreword by Bernard Rimland, Ph.D.

Wisconsin Institute of Nutrition, LLP
Milwaukee, Wisconsin
www.nutritioninstitute.com

FEAST WITHOUT YEAST: 4 STAGES TO BETTER HEALTH
Wisconsin Institute of Nutrition, LLP
http://www.nutritioninstitute.com

Cover design and graphic consultation: Tiffany Navins, Graphic Ingenuity
Book design: Lori Kornblum

Library of Congress Catalog in Publication Data:

Semon, Bruce, M.D., Ph.D., and Lori Kornblum
        Feast Without Yeast: 4 Stages to Better Health

        Includes Index
        1. Candida Related Complex. 2. Candida Diet - Recipes.
        3. Yeast Free Diet - Recipes. 4. Wheat/Gluten Free Diet - Recipes
        5. Milk/Casein Free Diet - Recipes 6. Allergy - Recipes
        7. Low Cholesterol - Recipes 8. Sugar Free Diet - Recipes
        9. Cookery (Natural Foods) 10. Cookery (Vegetarian)
        11. Cookery (Jewish)
Library of Congress Catalog Card Number: 99-93639
ISBN 0-9670057-0-1

                        10   9   8

To order single copies or to schedule Author appearances, or to schedule an appointment to see Dr. Semon contact us at: Wisconsin Institute of Nutrition, LLP, P.O. Box 170867, Milwaukee, WI 53217; Toll-Free in the U.S. and Canada: 1-877-332-7899.

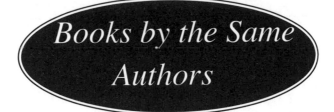

An Extraordinary Power to Heal (2003)
by Bruce Semon, M.D., Ph.D. and Lori Kornblum

.. .was written for people suffering from a wide range of supposedly untreatable medical conditions, ranging from Autism
to Chronic Fatigue Syndrome to Psoriasis. In every chapter, Dr.
Semon describes actual patients he has treated. *An Extraordinary
Power to Heal* goes further than *Feast Without Yeast* explaining why anti-yeast treatment works, and how the 4-Stages diet
works. He explains how yeast causes your immune system to
malfunction, causing illness instead of making you healthy. He
also explains how yeast-like chemicals found in food cause many
medical problems. *An Extraordinary Power to Heal* is written in
language everyone can understand, but scientifically documented
so health care practitioners can verify the basis for anti-yeast
treatment. *An Extraordinary Power to Heal* also includes dosing
information for nystatin, information about other medications
and supplements, suggestions for IEP (individualized education
plans) and a wealth of other information. *Feast Without Yeast* is
a practical introduction to anti-yeast treatment. *An Extraordinary
Power to Heal* gives you and your health care practitioner the
tools you need to understand and solve your health problems.

Extraordinary Foods for the Everyday Kitchen (2003)
by Lori Kornblum and Bruce Semon, M.D., Ph.D.

You will love our new cookbook, with more than 125 new, original **completely yeast free, gluten/wheat and casein/milk free
recipes** and more than 60 menus. We give tantalizing, easy new
recipes for tacos, pizza, salsa, falafel, salad dressings, mayonnaise, and other fabulous foods. *Extraordinary Foods* "offers a
mouth-watering spectrum of dishes . . . .[and] is a superb resource
for cooks who have to combine strict dietary requirements with
succulent taste in their epicurean creations." (*Wisconsin Book-
watch*, January 2004).

Who Should Use *Feast Without Yeast?*

You! When you answer "yes" to <u>any</u> of these 10 questions:

1. **Do you love good food? If "yes", you should use this book.** This cookbook is the one for you. Simply by eating delicious food that is free of toxic chemicals that can make you feel bad, you will feel great. What better reason to use a cookbook than to feel terrific after every meal? You can just skip to the recipes and ignore the nutritional information in the gray boxes in each recipe.

2. **Do you want to improve your general health? If yes, use this book.** Most people following the Four Stages **eliminate**:

   - sugar cravings
   - abdominal pain, bloating, and gas
   - headaches
   - diarrhea
   - constipation
   - general aches and pains

   Most people also **lose weight** and feel much **more energetic**.

3. **Are you looking for cholesterol-free food that tastes great? If "yes," use this book.** Look for the words "Cholesterol free" in the gray boxes in each recipe. Most of the recipes are cholesterol free, or can be made cholesterol free. Turn the page for more.......

4. **Are you a vegetarian? If "yes," you can eat all of the recipes** except in the chapter called Meat, Fish and Poultry. Many of the recipes are also vegan. For dairy free recipes, look for nutritional notes in the gray boxes in each recipe that say "Milk/casein free" and "Suitable through Stage III" and "Suitable through Stage IV." For egg free recipes, look for the words "Egg free."

5. **Do you cook kosher food? If "yes,"** you now have more than 225 additional recipes for your kitchen. Every recipe in the book is kosher. Just skip right to the recipes.

6. **Do you avoid artificial additives, preservatives and colorings? If "yes," you should use this book!** We use no artificial additives, preservatives, colorings, flavorings or other food enhancers. Just skip right to the recipes

7. **Do you like natural cooking? If "yes," try out our recipes.** We use whole grains, fresh fruits and vegetables, and almost no prepared ingredients. You will feel terrific after you eat what you have cooked.

8. **Looking for sugar free cooking? If "yes," you'll love this book.** We use no table sugar at all. Everything is sweetened naturally with unprocessed honey.

More on the next

page. . . .

9. **Are you allergic to common foods, such as milk, wheat, eggs, soy, rye or corn? If "yes," you should use this book.** We use no soy, rye or corn. Every recipe is safe for you. All recipes labelled in the gray boxes "Suitable through Stage III" or "Suitable through Stage IV" are free of milk and wheat. If eggs are a problem, look for "egg free" in the gray boxes.

10. **Do you suffer from any of these health conditions? If "yes" to any of these, you can benefit from this book.** Start at the beginning and follow

Headaches
Fatigue
Depression
Abdominal Pain
Bloating
Diarrhea
Constipation
Skin problems such
    as rashes, eczema,
    and psoriasis
Attention problems,
    including ADD
    and ADHD
Difficulty with con-
    centration
Confusion

Asthma
Autism
Rheumatoid Arthritis and
    other autoimmune
    diseases
Chronic vaginal yeast
    infections
Chronic ear infections
Abdominal Pain
Food allergies
Respiratory allergies
Eating disorders
Chemical Sensitivity
Chronic Fatigue Syndrome
Crohn's Disease
Fibromyalgia

This book is for <u>you</u>! So start cooking right here!

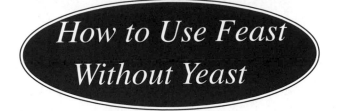

How to Use Feast Without Yeast

To use *Feast Without Yeast* as a regular cookbook, skip right to the recipes and start cooking. Ignore the information in the gray boxes.

For Cholesterol Free cooking, skip to the recipes and look for the words "Cholesterol free" in the gray boxes under the recipe title.

For Yeast Free cooking, start at the beginning of this book. Learn about the Four Stages and implement the diet, stage by stage. All recipes are free of yeast, mold and fermented foods. Each recipe in this cookbook is keyed to the Stages. Look at the information in the gray boxes under the recipe titles. Each recipe will say "Suitable through Stage..." If you are on Stage I, look for recipes suitable through Stage I, II, III or IV. If you are on Stage II, look for recipes suitable through Stage II, III or IV. If you are on Stage III, you can use recipes suitable through Stages III and IV. If you are on Stage IV, use recipes suitable through Stage IV.

For Wheat/Gluten and Milk/Casein Free cooking, look for the words "Wheat/gluten free" or "Milk/casein free" in the gray boxes under the recipe title, and look for the words "Suitable through Stage III" or "Suitable through Stage IV." The chapter called **The Four Stages** explains how to make the transition to a gluten and casein free life-style.

For Egg Free cooking, look for the words "Egg free" in the gray boxes under the recipe title.

For Vegetarian cooking, use all recipes other than **Meat, Fish and Poultry**.

For Kosher cooking, use all recipes.

This book is dedicated to our children,
Avi, Sarah and Mikah.

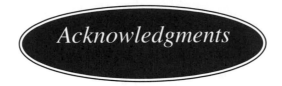

Acknowledgments

We would like to acknowledge the help of the many people who gave their time and effort to help us in writing this book: Dr. William Crook and Dr. Bernard Rimland, for their editorial comments and suggestions, encouragement and assistance; Dr. William Shaw, for his encouragement and assistance; our daughter Sarah, who invented and tested many of the recipes, who helped with the graphic design, and who just now is beginning to realize that there are hundreds of cookbooks in the world, not just ours; our many volunteer recipe testers, whose comments were invaluable in shaping this book: Dore Brown, Lisa Esmond, Nancy Harris, Linda Hoeppner, Betsy Kauffman, Candyce Kornblum, Charlene Kornblum, Carole O'Callaghan, Suzie Silbert, Anne Streicher; Emily and Robert Levine, for their technical assistance; Lorie O'Connor, for her insightful comments and proofreading; Cynthia Brown, for her editorial assistance and "real people" reminders; and of course, Dr. Semon's patients.

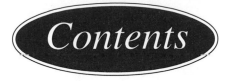

Contents

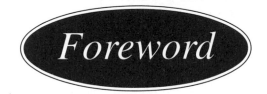

Foreword

This book will be a lifesaver for many families--families with as well as families without autistic children. Overwhelming evidence, much of it appearing in just the past few years, makes it superabundantly clear that a great many autistic children benefit enormously when certain foods are removed from their diets.

However, as the reader will soon learn, almost everyone, not just autistic children, is likely to enjoy improved health and vigor when problem-causing foods are identified and avoided. This book describes techniques, such as the simple expedient of reinstating the food to the diet after a period of avoidance, to confirm the value of the dietary changes.

A strong feature of this book is its emphasis upon the role that yeasts play in bringing about diet-related illness. While the authors include much information about solving the widely recognized problems caused in people sensitive to cow's milk and cereal grains, the authors perform a great additional service by providing compelling evidence to show that yeasts also can and do bring about much misery.

Let me tell you about an instructive personal experience. Some years ago my then-teenaged daughter Helen won a scholarship to a prestigious university in New York, to start the following September. Ordinarily a very bright, stable, confident and energetic person, Helen suddenly began to experience, in early August, bouts of extreme fatigue, headaches and confusion. She felt so "spacy" and disoriented that she was afraid to drive, fearing she would get lost or be involved in an accident.

My wife and I were very concerned. How could we let our daughter travel across the country and set up a residence in a strange city in her condition?

A psychologist friend suggested that Helen was suffering from anxiety, or phobias, due to her impending departure from home. "Nonsense!" I politely replied. "There is a physical cause, and we must find it."

I phoned my friend allergist Marshall Mandell, author of several books on unexpected consequences of food intolerances. After a few questions, Marshall honed in on Helen's summer job at a fish and chips cafe. At each table were plastic bottles full of vinegar that the patrons could use to flavor their fish and chips. One of Helen's duties was to make sure these bottles were filled.

Marshall suggested I provide Helen with a small bottle in which she could bring home a sample of the vinegar. He suggested that we pour the vinegar into a saucer and place it into a small enclosed space, such as a bathroom, then, after 10 or 15 minutes, ask Helen to walk into that room.

We followed Marshall's advice. Within a minute or two after entering the room, Helen emerged smiling. "That's it!" she said. "The fumes from the vinegar are causing my spacy feeling and headaches!"

Vinegar, it turns out, is produced by yeast and can be intoxicating to people who are sensitive to yeasts.

A sideline to the above story: Helen became so interested in food intolerances that she read all of Marshall's books and became an unpaid consultant to her friends with "psychological" problems.

One of these friends, a bright and vivacious young woman, became morose and depressed after starting a new job at a health food restaurant. Helen discovered that the young lady had fallen in love with the tuna, avocado and sprouts sandwiches, served on whole wheat bread, which were a favorite item on the menu. The young woman ate one sandwich herself every day. "Dr. Helen" prescribed, "no more tuna, avocado and sprouts sandwiches on whole wheat bread for two weeks," and "Bingo!" her friend soon returned to her vivacious personality. Her body was intolerant to at least one of the ingredients in the sandwich.

Quite apart from the above experience within my own family are the experiences that I have heard about from literally thousands of parents of autistic children over the past four decades.

Parents began writing to me, phoning me, and talking to me at conferences soon after my book *Infantile Autism* was published in 1964. I soon learned about many cases of children whose autism had cleared up remarkably when milk and/or wheat was removed from the child's diet.

The autistic daughter of an Air Force family became normal when the father was transferred to a base in northern Alaska and the family could not get cow's milk, but used reindeer milk instead! When then family returned to the U.S. and began serving their children cow's milk again, the daughter's autism quickly returned.

In her excellent book *Fighting for Tony*, nurse Mary Callahan told how her own son had been diagnosed as autistic by a number of specialists, but became normal when cow's milk was removed from his diet as a means of preventing his attacks of asthma. When the cow's milk was reinstated, both the asthma and the autism returned.

There are, in the files of the Autism Research Institute, many similar cases of autism due to wheat intolerance.

The role of yeasts as a cause of autism was first described by a California mother, Gianna Mayo, who noticed that her son's autism became worse during periods of damp weather, when he was exposed to more molds. She had read about yeast infections bringing about "mental" problems, and sought out a physician who would treat her autistic son with nystatin.

The *Los Angeles Times* published an account of Gianna Mayo's discovery in the early 1980's and immediately the Autism Research Institute began hearing from other parents who also found that their child's autism was in great part caused by yeasts.

The idea that yeasts can cause "mental" problems such as autism is not a popular one among most physicians. Sidney Baker, a Connecticut pediatrician who treats many autistic children, has encountered a great deal of skepticism among his medical colleagues. Sid likes to tell how he responds to such skepticism. He innocently asks, "Have you ever been in a liquor store?" His doctor friends look at him, startled. "Of course I've been in a liquor store. Why do you ask?" Sid continues: "Have you ever noticed all those bottles on liquor store shelves?" His doctor friends, now getting a bit concerned about Sid's sanity, or perhaps his sobriety, look even more puzzled. "Of course I've noticed the bottles. Why do you ask?" Sid responds, "Do you know what's in those bottles? I'll tell you: fungally-produced neurotoxins!"

Yes, it's true. Those bottles in the liquor store contain fungally-produced neurotoxins, in the form of alcohol. That is how liquor is made. And the person who has excess amounts of yeasts (fungi) in his or her system will produce alcohol-like substances that get into the blood stream and intoxicate the brain. (Sid told me, some years ago, that when he drives by a liquor store, he sees an imaginary sign over the door: **Fungally Produced Neurotoxins Sold Here**. A great idea!)

Well, now you know: each of us carries around in our gastrointestinal tract the site, or perhaps the future site, of a microbrewery which is capable of producing enough toxic chemicals to cause real problems, both mental and physical. This book provides you with the opportunity to make a giant stride toward preventing and treating that problem, as well as a host of other diet-related afflictions.

Bernard Rimland, Ph.D.
Autism Research Institute
San Diego, California
May, 1999

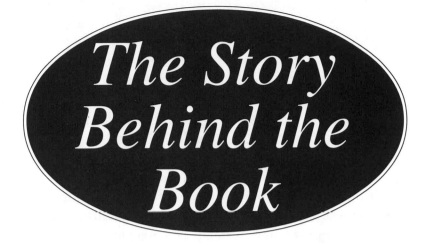

The Story Behind the Book

*Behind every book is a story. This is ours. We developed **Feast Without Yeast** based on our own experience trying to save our son's health. But we realized that it is a story that can and should be shared so that others may benefit from our experience. This chapter also covers the theoretical underpinnings of the Four Stages, and why **Feast Without Yeast** is unique among yeast free cookbooks.*

*F**east Without Yeast: Four Stages to Better Health* began on a Sunday morning in January, 1991, in Rockville, Maryland. Our four-and-a-half year old son was writhing on the floor screaming. He had been behaving this way on and off for six months, worse in the two months before this day. He had been to ten different doctors in the Washington, DC area, including some who were world renowned. None had been helpful. At age two he had been fine. From two-and-a-half to age four, his development had slowed down, but had not stopped. Starting a few days after his fourth birthday, he began to lose his speech. The speech loss started subtly, almost like a game. Avi would look at something for which he knew the words, then say, "I want. . .I want. . ." and I would fill in the name. He lost names of objects, names of colors, and words for common actions. Over the next six months, he went from losing words to being able to talk only in phrases he could pull out of his memory. His word for "car" was "let's get the car washed." His word for the Jewish holiday of Channukah was "in the days of the Macabees."

Avi also began to scream incessantly. He would scream blood curdling screams for hours at a time.

He was evaluated and placed in special education classes. During the first three weeks of class, he lost much of his speech, going from speaking in sentences to not being able to put two words together. He lost his toilet training, stopped eating and lost so much weight he went down two sizes. By this January day, our son could not use his hands. He walked around with them curled up. He sat in a swing spinning much of the day. He had lost all emotional contact except with his mother, and that was fleeting. We were under the care of a world famous psychiatrist, a psychologist, an occupational therapist and a speech therapist. We had seen three neurologists who subjected our son to countless tests, with negative results.   None of these experts could tell us what was happening to our angel. His younger sister, then only two, spent many hours trying to comfort her big brother, holding and hugging him as only a child can do.

It is difficult to put into words how a parent feels seeing their first-born son totally disintegrate into nothingness. He went from being a bright and able toddler to this writhing, screaming, little person, unable to talk, unable to communicate his wants, his needs or his love. The pain of the memories is real even eight years later. On this January day, he could say only a few words.

But on this early morning day there was to be an insight. I (Lori) was sitting up with Avi, as I had been each night for the previous month, during his waking hours of 2:00 to 7:00 AM. Avi was staring at something, saying "the lights, the lights." All of a sudden, it hit me: Avi was experiencing a migraine. He had had a peanut butter sandwich for bedtime snack, a food known to cause migraines, and this was it.

I (Bruce) grew up with a strong family history of migraines, and Lori suffered from them occasionally. Both of us experience what is called an "aura" before the pounding pain of the headache: flashing lights, dizzying patterns dancing before our eyes. My father had several migraines a week when he was in college, until he read an article in a magazine, stating that if one avoided certain foods, the migraines would decrease in frequency. This food avoidance became a family tradition. My father avoided these foods and his migraines diminished considerably. The magazine's list of foods to be avoided included such foods as chocolate, pickles, salad dressing, bacon, alcoholic beverages, nuts, and aged cheese. I have since seen from other headache clinics similar lists of foods to avoid. We decided to take away from Avi a small number of foods known to cause migraines.

We took away chocolate, peanut butter, orange juice, aged cheeses, and some other foods. The improvement was immediate. Avi looked and acted as if a weight had been lifted from his head. Only then could we see the onset of separate headaches, when we would make a mistake and give him foods we weren't supposed to, or when he would eat something that we learned later caused problems. We saw the headaches set in about three times a week instead of being chronic.

His symptoms of what we now know to be autism also began to diminish. He no longer screamed all the time. His behavior improved. He seemed more with us, more engagable. If he accidentally ate the wrong foods, the screaming began again. In the first few weeks, we noted that not all the screaming went away. We tried to determine what foods were still causing problems. At that time I was a research fellow at the National Cancer Institute, in a laboratory investigating links between nutrition and cancer.

Using the vast library of the National Institutes of Health, I began researching what might be causing Avi's problems. Based on my research, we decided to eliminate vinegar, a staple of our lives. Avi was a kid who ate ketchup on everything and loved Asian food, sprinkled with rice vinegar. Again, we saw immediate improvement, but knew that we were still missing something. I had no idea what the relationship was among the foods on the original list. Around this time, we also found that something in children's pain relievers was causing the headaches to last longer than usual. We do not know exactly what that substance is, suspecting many of the additives, including aspartame (NutraSweet) but do know that switching to pure acetaminophen (commonly known by the brand name of Tylenol), and later to pure ibuprofen (commonly known by the brand names of Motrin and Advil), shortened the life of the headaches. Life for Avi improved considerably, but he still suffered tremendous pain and still continued to lose his speech. Avi's speech disappeared totally in March, 1991. He uttered no real words for five years.

We got our next break about eight weeks later with the Jewish holiday of Passover. For this holiday, all foods containing yeast, leavening and fermented foods are eliminated. This holiday lasts eight days. Three days into Passover, our son was clearly improving again. He appeared much more comfortable. By this time his speech was gone, so we were dependent on how he looked and behaved. His behavior had improved to the point that he was accepted into a special education speech and language summer program.

After those eight days, though, Avi deteriorated. The screaming intensified. We had no idea what had happened. What was in the food that we were now giving again? We had many snack foods from the health food store, all supposedly healthy. I (Bruce) read the labels and the one ingredient that I did not recognize was barley malt. What was this substance?

After some investigation, I found out that barley malt is a raw material used in making beer. The malt is made from a specially grown barley. The barley is allowed to sprout under controlled conditions. After a certain period of time, the sprouted barley is heated. The resulting substance is called malt and is the raw material for making beer. The malt is also sweet and is sold as a sugar substitute.

In beer manufacture, yeast is mixed with the malt and chemically alters the malt to form alcohols and many other chemicals. This process is called fermentation.

Why is malt such a problem? I pursued my investigation over the years and was able to obtain from a beer manufacturer a list of chemicals found in barley malt. Many of these chemicals are toxic and affect the nervous system. Many slow the brain down, which may be part of the reason these chemicals and malt are so bad for children with developmental and behavioral problems. This information made sense. I had observed clinically that the behavior of even neurologically typical children can deteriorate when they eat foods containing malt. Our ten year old daughter, for example, becomes a typical whiny, demanding, unhappy preadolescent a few hours after she eats malted foods. She has become so aware of how ill she feels when she eats malt that she reads labels before eating anything unfamiliar. About a month after we took away malt from Avi's diet, a baby-sitter unwittingly gave him two bowls of cereal with malt. We came home from a walk and found Avi sitting on the couch, staring into space. He remained in that trance like state for ten days. Fortunately, we have never had that experience again.

Besides the malt, what was the relationship among the items on the list? Vinegar is literally spoiled wine, which is a fermented product. But what about chocolate and nuts? I went back to my research to find out. I knew about certain cancer causing chemicals in food. One is called aflatoxin, a potent cancer-causer found in small amounts in peanuts. Aflatoxin comes from a fungus, called Aspergillus, which contaminates the peanut plant. Chocolate beans are dried with a fungus. Now the relationship among the items on the migraine headache list became clear. Except for malt, all of the foods on the list were products of yeast fermentation or of fungus contamination. Yeast and fungus have many similar biochemical pathways, although in general, fungi produce poisons much more potent than yeast can produce. Even though malt is not a direct product of fermentation, I found some overlap in the chemicals produced during the formation of malt and the products of fermentation. Some of the chemicals found in malt are also found in chocolate and coffee.

I concluded that something produced by yeast and fungus was wreaking havoc on our son. We needed to know what it was. My lab happened to be practically next door to the U.S. Army germ warfare labs. Several people there work in specialized fermentation. One such set of people was right down the hall. They got me started on my research.

The first chemical I found that I thought might be causing a problem is called acetol. Acetol is a skin irritant and an eye irritant (probably known from research to see if it could be used in cosmetics). Acetol is in vinegar. Acetol is also found in maple syrup. I thought I was making progress. The identification of what foods could cause problems for our son was becoming easier. As I identified what foods contain which chemicals and we took these foods away, Avi improved, albeit slowly.

We ran into another problem at this time. People like fermented foods. They taste good. Barley malt and vinegar are very common additives in foods. Vinegar has a zesty taste. Barley malt is apparently cheaper than sugar and is sold as a sugar substitute. Barley malt is also promoted as a "grain sweetener" in health food stores, an alternative to refined sugar. My (Lori) shopping tours to the grocery stores began to take on the nature of a research experiment in itself. Vinegar is the staple of all commercially produced condiments: ketchup, mustard, mayonnaise, salsa, salad dressing and many sauces. Avi's favorite foods used to be soy hot dogs with ketchup, mustard, salsa and mayonnaise. Barley malt seems to be baked into nearly everything, including bread, bagels, breakfast cereal and many health food snacks. It is in so-called natural chocolates and candies instead of sugar. Barley malt is even in many commercial white flours, so even home-baked goods were suspect. We found we could no longer buy most commercially prepared foods. We had to prepare almost all our own food, and we had to devise new ways to prepare that food. Our days of Hot and Sour Soup were over for good.

Once we eliminated barley malt and all other malted products (maltodextrin, malted barley flour, and so on), vinegar, and yeast, the improvement was dramatic. We began to see the light at the end of the tunnel, but little did we know how long that tunnel was. Reaching the end of the tunnel is still a goal, although after eight years, we are much closer. Eight years ago, simply decreasing Avi's headaches to once a week or once every two weeks, and seeing his behavior improve and his autistic symptoms decrease were major victories. We had turned the tide before we lost Avi altogether. He was coming back to us, very, very slowly. It took two more years, and much more experimentation, to completely eliminate Avi's debilitating headaches. Another two years of experimentation eliminated Avi's eczema and itching.

W e began this cookbook around that time, although we did not intend to write a cookbook for other people. We needed to write down the recipes that we created that our family enjoyed eating, so we could recreate them and let other people cook for our children. *Feast Without Yeast* is the culmination of eight years of effort at trying to come up with good tasting food without using anything fermented. As we removed more foods from our son's diet, we created more recipes. For us, developing such recipes has been an absolute necessity because our son has remained sensitive to any fermented food, is allergic to corn, soy, eggs, wheat and milk, and does not tolerate gluten. We wanted to keep our son healthy and still eat what he calls great tasting food.

We found, though, that foods were not the only key to Avi's puzzle. Around April of 1991, after that first Passover holiday, one of the many health care professionals we were seeing suggested we look at an outstanding book called *The Yeast Connection* by Dr. William Crook. Dr. Crook compiled treatment histories of people who have problems with something called *Candida albicans*, a type of fungus which at times resembles yeast. We found that Dr. Crook recommended eliminating many of the foods we had found to be problematic for Avi, although there were some very significant differences at that time. Could it be that Avi had a yeast problem? Certainly no professional had ever mentioned this, but certainly no health care professional had been able to help us to this point. At that time, there was not a reliable test for systemic *Candida* infection, as there is now. * We decided to try treating Avi with a nontoxic medication called nystatin. Nobody, including the doctor who had introduced us to this concept, would prescribe nystatin for us. Fortunately, I had a medical license.

Within a few days of starting on the nystatin, Avi made a year's growth in playground development. He got off the swings, where he usually spent his hours of playground time. He began climbing jungle gyms, sliding down slides, and beginning to look like a four year old kid again. Avi still did not get his speech back, but he was beginning to be able to function.

M y research continued. I realized that eliminating certain foods and treating the yeast *Candida albicans* are two pieces of the same puzzle. I found the following basic principles of anti-yeast treatment :

The yeast *Candida albicans* is a normal resident inside of our intestine and colon. This yeast can also be found at times in the mouth and in the vagina. Sometimes this yeast overgrows and the doctor recognizes this overgrowth of yeast as a yeast infection of the vagina, or in the mouth, where this infection is commonly called thrush.

Bacteria also reside inside the intestine, sharing space with the yeast. After the use of antibiotics to kill bacteria, the yeast grow

---

*Dr. William Shaw has developed a urine organic acids test for the metabolites of yeast. This test is available from him through the Great Plains Laboratory, 9335 W. 75th Street, Overland Park, KS 66204. See his website at www.greatplainslaboratory.com, or call his lab at (913) 341-8949. Individuals can order the test kit, but a doctor must prescribe the test.

to fill in the space left by the bacteria's removal. Even after the antibiotics have been stopped, the yeast continue to grow at a higher level, making their toxic chemical compounds. Major increases in hormones, such as during pregnancy and while using birth control pills, can also encourage yeast growth.

Yeast make a number of chemical compounds which the body picks up and absorbs. These compounds are mildly toxic to most people, who may not feel much effect. Other people may have more effect, including vaginal yeast infections or diarrhea. Still other people, however, have much more trouble handling these compounds and they may feel sick, although neither they nor their doctors generally have any idea why. These toxic compounds can cause many symptoms, ranging from diarrhea or constipation to depression. Yeast can cause other problems by other mechanisms, including skin conditions such as eczema and psoriasis, autoimmune disorders such as rheumatoid arthritis, and multiple sclerosis. These disorders can be treated using the same anti-yeast diet and medications.

I have treated many people for many of these disorders. I have found in my practice that the best way to reverse the problems that yeast create is to take the anti-yeast drug nystatin and to remove fermented foods from the diet. This approach kills the yeast in the body and keeps more toxic chemicals from being introduced into the body through foods. Nystatin kills the yeast living in the intestine. Then the yeast can no longer make the toxic chemical compounds. Because nystatin, unlike some other antifungals, is not absorbed into the body, Nystatin is not harmful. Nystatin has no long term side effects listed in the physicians' guides to medications such as the *Physicians' Desk Reference*.

Removing harmful foods from the diet prevents more toxic chemicals from being introduced into the body. Yeast and fungi make antibacterial compounds. Fermented foods in the diet contain antibacterial compounds. These antibacterial compounds will bring the yeast back if these foods, such as vinegar and barley malt, are not removed from the diet. Such foods also contain toxic yeast compounds. For the nystatin to work, the diet must be changed to restrict such fermented foods.

A lthough it seemed at first that the diet recommended in *The Yeast Connection* could have saved us a lot of work, and perhaps would have saved Avi's speech had we discovered the book sooner, we found that it did not answer the questions that Avi posed to us. Had we followed that diet, which at the time was the standard for anti-yeast diets, Avi still would have been eating many of the foods that we know cause him tremendous problems.

The main difference between the diet that I developed and diets based on *The Yeast Connection* is in the meat versus carbo-hydrate content of the diets. Diets based on *The Yeast Connection* contain a great deal of meat and recommend eliminating most carbohydrates. One can find this idea's genesis in the pioneering work of Dr. Orian Truss, in *The Missing Diagnosis.* Dr. Truss postulated that because, experimentally, *Candida albicans* grows well in carbohydrate and not particularly well in protein, one should remove carbohydrate so that the yeast doesn't grow as well. The main recommendation growing out of Dr. Truss' work has been to limit carbohydrate and yeast from bread and substitute more meat and fish.

In my practice, however, I find that the human body is not as simple as a test tube nor is the human diet as simple as culture media for yeast in a petri plate.

I have treated many frustrated patients who have followed the recommendations to eliminate sugar and bread from their diets, and to increase meat and fish. These patients enjoyed few results. Their symptoms include autism, chronic fatigue syndrome, arthritis, fibromyalgia, multiple sclerosis, skin conditions and many more. The reason for their lack of results is not their lack of effort, but the fact that the main dietary yeast offenders (vinegar and barley malt) had been left in their diets. In fact, most of the anti-yeast and allergy related cookbooks have vinegar as a staple food and recommend a diet high in animal protein and nuts, which are thoroughly mold contaminated. Even diets that eliminate vinegar tend to use apple juice concentrate as a sweetener, which is high in chemicals toxic to people who are sensitive to yeast.

Our experience with our son and with my other patients is that this dietary recommendation of high protein and low carbohydrate does not help many people. When yeast spoils meat, the toxic chemicals formed are worse than those formed by yeast in carbohydrate. In addition, chicken and pigs are fed cottonseed meal which is contaminated with a fungus called *Aspergillus*. I speculate that the animals store the *Aspergillus* poisons in their fat. This technique is a common way for animals to handle poisons. It is possible that storing the fungus poisons is one reason why yeast sensitive patients should not eat large amounts of meat. Meat from the right sources and in small quantities is acceptable on the anti-yeast diet, however. We have found that the easiest meats to eat are veal and lamb, which is consistent with recommendations of allergists. Cows receive less or no cottonseed meal (other feeds are cheaper) and there is little time for any poisons to accumulate in the calf prior to slaughter. We have included a few veal and lamb recipes in this cookbook. We found with our son and again with many patients since that a diet of complex carbohydrate is the best for yeast problems.

Another major difference between my approach and the approach in other anti-yeast treatment and cookbooks is that I recommend a food removal (elimination) diet rather than a rotation diet. The principle behind a rotation diet is that the body can tolerate a certain amount of problematic food if it is not introduced very often. A patient is put on a schedule where certain foods are eaten in certain combinations, at certain times and on certain days. I have not found rotation diets to be very effective and from personal experience, have found them to be very difficult to implement.

The principle behind an elimination diet is that the foods themselves cause toxic reactions, and one does not want to introduce toxins into the body at any time. Although the elimination diet takes some adjustment in the beginning, the diet is easier to implement in the long run because we introduce the eliminations gradually in stages, which are easier to remember in the long run. In addition, we have found that by going slowly and gradually, the patient finds just the right level of foods to eliminate. We explain all of this in the chapters, *The Four Stages: Your Path to Better Health* and *The Four Stages for Children*.

I left the National Cancer Institute in August of 1991. A month later I began treating patients for *Candida albicans* using the dietary principles I developed while working with our son and using the nontoxic anti-yeast drug nystatin. I found that I could treat supposedly untreatable conditions such as autism, psoriasis, eczema, chronic fatigue syndrome, multiple sclerosis, chronic vaginal yeast infections, attention deficit disorder, chronic ear infections, and refractory depression. These conditions all respond to treatment of *Candida albicans*.

I usually tell patients that in treating yeast about one third of the treatment response is from changing diet and two thirds is from taking nystatin. However, very little response is seen from nystatin alone if the diet is not changed. Changing the diet is most important in problems such as headaches, skin problems and abdominal pain. For other conditions mentioned above, changing diet gives a partial response. Nonetheless, the partial response may be beneficial and may give one the encouragement to find a doctor who will prescribe nystatin.

Feast Without Yeast, then, is the culmination to this point of our experience as parents, and my experience as a physician. It is mostly vegetarian, based on complex carbohydrates and whole foods. We do not use exotic grains, as we have not had much luck with them. We do not use exotic meats (we keep Kosher and this book is Kosher). We use no fillers, substitutes, additives, preservatives, or chemicals of any type. We use no corn, soy, or rye products. Only one prepared food is recommended, a brand of rice pasta, because it is a great food! Even the most yeast sensitive children and adults can rely on any of the recipes in this book, which, in combination with medical treatment for *Candida albicans* with the anti-yeast drug nystatin, will treat yeast successfully in almost everyone.

One question remained for us: why did our son continue to suffer from periodic bouts of eczema and hives? Part of the problem lay in attempting to liberalize the diet. He turned out also to have sensitivities to wheat, milk and eggs, like many other children who suffer from autism. I went back to the library and found that milk and wheat contain substances that are toxic to the brains of sensitive people. Thus, we began working on another series of recipes, these containing no gluten (the part of wheat that causes the food sensitivities), casein (the protein in milk causing the food sensitivities) or eggs.

After eliminating all of these foods, we are left with what seems like little, but turns out to be the basis of a rich, flavorful and extremely healthy diet: beans, rice, potatoes, tomatoes, fresh berries, safflower oil, sea salt, honey, fresh vegetables, lemons and herbs. But even with those limited foods we have developed many very tasty recipes which our guests love to eat.

Because **Feast Without Yeast** is mostly vegetarian, most of the recipes contain no cholesterol. However, this book is not a catch-all fad diet book. You will find many recipes contain a liberal amount of salt to flavor foods like beans that themselves have little flavor. We also use safflower oil, which is cholesterol free, and butter in sufficient quantity to add flavor to food. Do not be fooled by individual recipes, though! Following this diet overall has resulted in our own family's lower cholesterol and lower blood pressure because in the overall context of the diet, the additional salt and fat do not cause health problems.

Many people ask us whether this treatment has been a "cure" for our son. We cannot say that it has been, but we cannot say that it has not been. Avi still does not talk, but talking is not the only important part of life. Avi now is able to relate to people emotionally. He is out of pain. This treatment has been the foundation of a better life for Avi. Without dietary intervention and nystatin, Avi could not have benefitted from any other treatment. He is in school in an integrated setting, a regular school and a regular classroom, with an aide, and has been since first grade. He could not tolerate the presence of other children before starting on this diet. He could not tolerate being touched. Now Avi loves tickles, hugs and touches, even from strangers. Avi has benefitted from an intensive in-home applied behavioral analysis program, again, which he could not have tolerated without the diet and nystatin treatment. Avi still does not talk fluently, but has regained some speech. Avi is a far cry from the little boy spinning on the swing with his hands curled up, looking at nobody, caring for nothing, screaming all the time. He is a happy and healthy child, free of extraordinary pain, and able to function much better socially and emotionally in the world.

We hope that you will use *Feast Without Yeast* as your guide to better health. We have found that most people who follow this diet, in conjunction with treatment from a sensitive health care practitioner, enjoy much better health. We caution you not to start or stop any medication without consulting your physician. If you have questions about how this diet will affect your health, please consult a health care practitioner who is knowledgeable about your health and about treating yeast problems. We cannot promise you results, because everyone's body is different, but we can promise you that you will be able to make delicious food for you and your family, and you do not need to reinvent the wheel. So start here and take the first step toward improving your health.

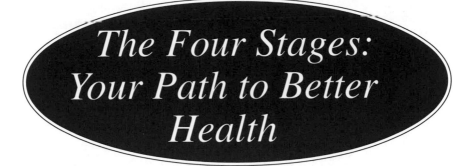

The Four Stages: Your Path to Better Health

Feast Without Yeast is your guide to changing your life-style to promote better health. We give you a step by step approach to changing your diet, which you should follow gradually to make the process natural and easy. Many people need not make drastic changes to begin feeling better. In this chapter, you will find:

~ *Good Health: The First Resort*

~ *Changing Your Diet to Improve Your Health*

~ *Implementing Change Slowly and Gradually*

~ *Introducing the Four Stages*

~ *Ready, Set, Go: Stage I*

> *Most people can stop here! But, for those who continue to need treatment. . . .*

~ *Moving on: Stage II*

> *Most people moving on to Stage II stop here. But, for people who need more . . .*

~ *Removing gluten and casein: Stage III*

> *Only a few people will need to move on to Stage IV. . . .*

~ *The Final Step: Stage IV*

~ *The Lists in one Place*

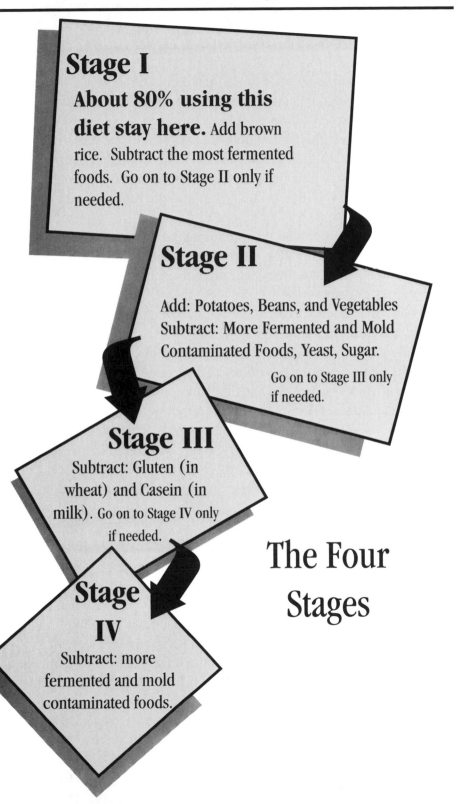

Stage I

About 80% using this diet stay here. Add brown rice. Subtract the most fermented foods. Go on to Stage II only if needed.

Stage II

Add: Potatoes, Beans, and Vegetables
Subtract: More Fermented and Mold Contaminated Foods, Yeast, Sugar.

Go on to Stage III only if needed.

Stage III
Subtract: Gluten (in wheat) and Casein (in milk). Go on to Stage IV only if needed.

Stage IV
Subtract: more fermented and mold contaminated foods.

The Four Stages

Good Health: the First Resort

Feast Without Yeast is more than a cookbook; it is a life-style book. We give you a plan for making dietary changes that we hope will improve your overall health, and recipes to help you implement those changes. This plan is concrete and easy to follow. Instead of giving you general advice, and leaving the particulars to your imagination, we give you specific lists to follow. . . .both the foods you <u>can</u> eat and the foods you should not eat.

Improving your health by changing what you eat can seem to be a very challenging task. Most people only try dietary change as a last resort because they fear not being able to eat everything that looks or tastes good.

So why should you do it?

The reason is simple: you will feel better. The yeast which is found in bread is called *Saccharomyces*. This is the same yeast that ferments alcoholic beverages. This yeast makes chemicals which affect many people, causing such problems as headaches, fatigue and depression. Chemicals found in the common food additive barley malt cause these same kinds of problems.

In addition, there is another type of yeast found in the intestinal tract (the gut) called *Candida albicans*. While the presence of yeast is considered normal for some people, your body does not make this yeast. Your body simply allows the yeast to have a place to live and grow. *Candida albicans* makes many of the same chemicals as the yeast in bread.

So, your body has yeast living inside the intestinal tract and you take in yeast and chemicals from the food you eat. You need to attack the problem from both sides: inside your body and from the outside, from your diet. This joint attack will help to eliminate the chemicals or toxins that are making you feel sick.

Feast Without Yeast helps you attack the yeast and chemicals you take in from your food, which in turn helps limit the amount of yeast living inside your body.

Changing your diet, that is, changing the food you eat, and using the recipes in this cookbook, helps to reduce the yeast you take in from the outside. This in turn helps to reduce intestinal yeast because the yeast you take in from your food helps the intestinal yeast to grow. Eliminating the yeast from your diet restricts the ability of the intestinal yeast to grow.

For example, in laboratory tests, the intestinal yeast *Candida albicans* grows very well in malt, which is one of the main foods you need to eliminate.

Why are these chemicals so bad for you?

Many of the chemicals yeast produce are made to kill bacteria. If you continue to eat foods which yeast have produced, such as vinegar (vinegar is literally spoiled wine), you are taking in a low level of antibacterial chemicals all the time. Another name for antibacterial chemicals is antibiotics.

Antibacterial chemicals kill bacteria. They kill both good and bad bacteria. Because yeast and bacteria both live in the gut, killing the bacteria provides space for the yeast already present in the gut to grow. This creates an imbalance between the yeast and the bacteria. The bacteria killed are not necessarily bad (such as the bacteria that cause disease).

When the yeast take up the space meant for bacteria, the good bacteria cannot recolonize and grow. The imbalance gets worse instead of better, and many people suffer health problems because of it.

Taking in antibacterial chemicals favors the growth of yeast and favors the continuation of all the problems which yeast cause. Using *Feast Without Yeast* makes it harder for yeast to grow in the intestinal tract.

Now you can understand how *Feast Without Yeast* will help you approach dietary change as a first resort. You will find that you can eat great tasting food and feel good, too.

I recommend changing your diet as a first resort because it has tremendous health benefits without the adverse side effects, of medications. I know this from clinical experience.

There are many psychiatric and medical conditions that I know from clinical experience will respond to dietary change. In my own psychiatric practice, I will prescribe conventional medication when the patient wishes to use medication instead of using diet to attack their problems. However, many of these medications have debilitating side effects, and may not as effective as dietary change in relieving the symptoms. Dietary change has no negative side effects other than inconvenience.

This chapter covers the general steps to changing your diet. Because changing childrens' diets presents special challenges, we deal with those challenges in greater detail in the chapter called *The Four Stages for Children*. Read *The Four Stages for Children* after you have read this chapter.

Changing Your Diet to Improve Your Health

My clinical experience has taught me that the people who change their diets experience lasting health benefits. The only side effect of changing one's diet is inconvenience. Most patients who follow this diet experience more energy, being able to make major life changes, and eliminating health problems that brought the patient to me.

These conditions have included headaches, autism, attention deficit disorder and attention deficit hyperactivity disorder, fibromyalgia, depression, multiple sclerosis, rheumatoid arthritis, chronic fatigue syndrome, uncontrolled eczema and psoriasis, and other health problems.

We give you step-by-step method to change your diet, and more than 200 recipes to help you implement these changes. At first, this method may appear complicated. However, it actually is easy to follow once you start using it.

We are the first to recognize, though, that changing diet presents social and emotional difficulties for everyone, including family.

Food has social and emotional implications as well as nutritional value. We often say, if we didn't live with the doctor, we would have a much harder time sticking with the program.

To change diet, you need to have a good enough reason to override these social and emotional difficulties. What better reason than giving someone the opportunity to live a better life?

Untreated or ineffectively treated illness is at least equally as inconvenient as cooking a few special meals. In our own lives, before we found that diet related to our son's autism, we had night after night of screaming and staying awake from 2:00 AM until 7:00 AM. This affected the entire family for months. We know when our son gets into something he should not eat. The insomnia, discomfort and general difficulties reemerge.

Certainly taking a few extra steps to cook good food beats that! Changing diet is relatively easy compared with a life in agony.

I have had patients come to me with such severe itching that their lives were intolerable; with tingling pain in their hands and feet; with migraine headaches, and with other conditions that did not respond well to conventional medical treatment.

To my knowledge, changing diet, and adding an anti-yeast medication called nystatin, significantly helped all of those who followed the diet. For some conditions, including autism, changing diet and using nystatin has been much more effective in producing lasting change in people than many of the medications I commonly prescribe in my psychiatric practice.

You do not need to take nystatin to feel better, though. Changing diet will help some people immensely. Even for the most difficult cases, which do benefit from nystatin, dietary change accounts for at least a third of health improvement.

So jump right in and start now!

The tragedy in waiting to decide about whether you are ready to tackle this diet is that intervention is best done as soon as possible. There is no such concept as "premature" in deciding to use diet to tackle complex health problems.

Key Thought: Do not stop any current medication based on this book. You must consult with your doctor. Dietary change will not affect any medication.

Implementing Change Slowly and Gradually

The first step in any major life change is to implement the change slowly and gradually. You don't learn to swim by jumping off the diving board! You need to learn new habits, find new foods to eat, and different ways to cook, which takes time.

We analogize this dietary change to a series of steps, or stages—platforms to which you will ascend, stay for a time, and see if your health is better. If so, you stay. If not, you go on to the next stage.

Although there are four stages altogether, about 90 percent of my patients only need to go to Stages I or II to reap the health benefits of this new life-style. In fact, some people can reach the platform of good health from the first step, Stage I-A, and need not go on to Stage I-B.

Others need to go to the next Stage, I-B. Still more need to go to the next stage, Stage II. There is a small group that will need to proceed to Stage III. The highest step of all, Stage IV, is only for the most sensitive people.

More than eighty percent of the recipes in ***Feast Without Yeast*** are suitable for Stage IV, the last stage. Every recipe "suitable through Stage IV" is also suitable for Stages I, II and III.

We urge you not to rush yourself to Stage IV too soon. Even if you love challenges and want to start with Stage IV, restrain yourself. Most people will not end up at Stage IV. Starting at Stage IV will deprive you of many foods that you may be able to eat. You don't want to lose that opportunity! In addition, going from a "normal" American diet to Stage IV is too drastic for most families, including my own. You will end up failing because you simply cannot enforce the diet. You will have much more success implementing the diet over the course of several months in a way that enables you to stick with it.

Key Thought: This cookbook is intended to be a companion to medical treatment, not a substitute. I recommend seeing a health care practitioner experienced in implementing yeast free diets and gluten/casein free diets, who can also treat the underlying yeast problem medically. As you begin to implement a yeast free diet, you may also be treated with nystatin, an antifungal medication. Follow your health care practitioner's advice.

Introducing the Four Stages

The Basic Principles

The Four Stages are about better health. By taking out of your diet foods that are bad for your health, and introducing foods that are good for your health, you will experience positive changes in your body. The Four Stages are not about fad dieting. In fact, some aspects of the four stages may surprise you.

We do not follow the currently fashionable notion that healthy diets use no fat or salt. In moderation, good fat (safflower oil) and sea salt actually are good for your health.

The yeast free diet is low in animal protein, so some added fat is necessary to make you feel full (satiety) and to flavor the food. Safflower oil is good for you in a positive way, containing all of the essential fatty acids. Sea salt is a good flavor enhancer and contains lots of minerals. Unless you know that salt causes you adverse health effects, use the salt in these recipes.

Many of the foods eliminated on this diet are flavorful and have nutritional benefits for people who are not sensitive to yeast. However, those foods are toxic, meaning poisonous, to yeast sensitive people. *Feast Without Yeast* presents a balance between eating good tasting food and keeping healthy.

In our family, on Stage IV, we rely heavily on foods fried in safflower oil, such as potatoes (hash browns, french fries) and fried beans. These foods satisfy the hunger, taste and some of the nutritional needs of growing children who eat mostly beans and rice.

Children who have been following Stage IV, even with all of the fried foods, tend to be healthy and not have weight problems, because the overall diet is low in fat and healthy. You have a broad range of choice of recipes and foods to find combinations that satisfy your family.

You may discover that people in your family may have certain food intolerances in addition to yeast sensitivity, just as we have. For example, this book does not contain tofu recipes, because our family does not tolerate soy products. This intolerance is not yeast related. If your family tolerates soy, tofu is a good substitute for meat or other foods that you have removed. If you discover other food intolerances, eliminate those foods as well.

An overview

Now that you are prepared to help yourself and your family improve your health, and now that you know the basics behind the Four Stages, you are ready to begin. Each Stage has foods that you should add, and refers you to a chapter called ***Shopping Lists*** so you can see the wide variety of foods you continue to be able to eat. Then, each stage has a list of foods to remove. We provide these lists as you go through this chapter. You will also find all of the lists together at the end of the chapter.

We also have coded every recipe in *Feast Without Yeast* to the Stages. Look at the gray box under each recipe title. "Suitable through Stage I" means only people on Stage I can use these recipes safely. "Suitable through Stage II" means that people on Stages I and II can use these recipes safely. "Suitable through Stage III" means that people using Stages I, II or III can use these recipes. "Suitable through Stage IV" means the recipes are suitable for everyone.

Stage I is the first stage.   About 80 percent of my patients are so successful, meaning that they feel so well, on Stage I that they need not proceed any further.

This stage takes only a few days for some people, but takes a few weeks for others.

We have divided Stage I into two parts, Stage I-A and Stage I-B. Stage I-A introduces and begins to implement yeast free living by adding brown rice and removing the most fermented and problematic foods from your diet. These foods are concentrated sources of dietary toxins.

Stage I-B removes more fermented foods. All of the recipes in this cookbook are suitable for Stage I-A, and most are suitable for Stage I-B.

If you still are not feeling well, you may not be among the 80 percent who can stay at Stage I. You should continue to Stage II.

Stage II adds potatoes and beans, and introduces some different types of food, including yeast free bread. Stage II removes some more fermented foods, including yeasted bread. Go to this stage after a few weeks of Stage I, if you or your child still are not feeling "100 percent." Nearly all of the recipes in this cookbook are suitable for Stage II.

About 90 percent of people will feel so well on the combination of Stages I and II that they will not need to go any further. However, if you feel that your health needs more attention, continue to Stage III.

Stage III introduces another concept, living without gluten. Gluten is a protein found in wheat, barley, rye, oats and some other grains. Stage III also takes casein out of the diet. Casein is a protein found in milk. Large numbers of people who are yeast sensitive also are sensitive to gluten and casein. Transitioning to a milk/casein and wheat/gluten free diet is not exceptionally difficult. You can eat all of the foods on Shopping Lists 1 and 2 from the chapter called *Shopping Lists*. Substitute rice and potatoes, and follow the more than 175 recipes in *Feast Without Yeast* that are labelled "Suitable through Stage III" or "Suitable through Stage IV."

More than eighty percent of the recipes in this book are designed for people sensitive to yeast, gluten and casein. Look for the recipe designation "Wheat/Gluten Free" and "Milk/Casein Free."

Stage IV is the last, most restrictive, stage. Only a few people--probably 5 out of every 100--go on to Stage IV. I find, however, that many people with autism as well as many people with skin problems need to experiment with this stage.

Your diet can be rich with a variety of tastes and textures. More than four fifths of the recipes in this book can be used for Stage IV. We have followed Stage IV for many years and have served entire meals to company that were Stage IV meals. Our guests frequently have commented on how good they feel after eating at our table.

Ready, Set, Go: Stage I

Stage I is the first step toward changing your health. We divide Stage I into two parts, Stage I-A and Stage I-B. Begin at the beginning, with Stage I-A, go slowly. If you are comfortable on Stage I-A, but still are experiencing health problems, proceed to Stage I-B.

The first step is to see what you can eat, not what you can't. The Stage I list of allowable foods is on page 37. To help you shop, look at *Shopping Lists* (pages 95-98). Copy pages 96-98

(Lists 1, 2 and 3) and take them to the store. You will have the basics of all of the recipes in this book if you stock up on the items on those lists.

You can eat everything on those lists--which is quite a lot. You should keep in mind while you are removing foods from your diet all of the foods that you can add, all of the new recipes you can try, and how much better you will feel. You should budget extra time to go shopping at this point, because you need to really scrutinize labels.

In the first week or so, you will add brown rice to your diet, and should begin experimenting with recipes that use rice. We have a chapter devoted to recipes that are *Mainly Rice*.

You also will remove the most fermented and problematic foods in your diet. These foods are concentrated sources of dietary toxins.

I have found in practice that the majority of people benefit so much from this stage that they need not eliminate any other foods.

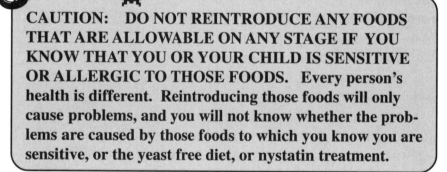

CAUTION: DO NOT REINTRODUCE ANY FOODS THAT ARE ALLOWABLE ON ANY STAGE IF YOU KNOW THAT YOU OR YOUR CHILD IS SENSITIVE OR ALLERGIC TO THOSE FOODS.   Every person's health is different. Reintroducing those foods will only cause problems, and you will not know whether the problems are caused by those foods to which you know you are sensitive, or the yeast free diet, or nystatin treatment.

I have had more than one patient who has looked at the list for Stage I-A and concluded that they could safely add back foods that they knew caused bad reactions, because we did not recommend removing those foods at this stage. The two main groups of food that seem to cause the most problems are dairy products and corn containing products.

I had one parent, for example, who knew that her child had a problem with milk and cheese. She added those items back into her child's diet because Stage I does not eliminate milk and cheese. Her child then experienced tremendous problems, which the parent blamed on a reaction to killing yeast called "die off," or on nystatin, but which more than likely had been caused by the milk and cheese.

Other patients who have been doing relatively well have added corn back into their diet, or have increased corn, and have had bad reactions, or have seen lack of progress.

Avoid these pitfalls!

Stay on Stage I-A for at least a week. You can stay on Stage I-A for a longer time. This is your chance to get adjusted to dietary change, try out some new recipes, and begin to feel better.

When you are ready, or when your health care practitioner advises you to do so, move on to Stage I-B.

Stage I-A gets at the foods that are the most fermented and the most mold contaminated. The most important foods to eliminate are vinegar and barley malt.

Why these two?

I (Bruce) have found, in my clinical experience, that eliminating those two has the most immediate impact on health and behavior.

Barley malt is a product that starts with the grain barley. The barley is specially sprouted, then heated. This heated product becomes the raw material for making beer. Barley malt is found in many cereals, crackers, breads, white flour and bagels and in many health food snacks. Although barley malt is the worst offender, other types of malt, including maltodextrin (usually malt added to corn syrup), also cause harm. When shopping read labels carefully and avoid anything with the word "malt" in it.

You will be amazed at how many commercially prepared foods contain "malt," "barley malt," "maltodextrin," or "malted barley flour."

Malt is in bagels, for example. So on Stage I-A, you must eliminate bagels. Malt is also in nearly all commercially processed white flour. So even home baking does not guarantee you are malt free. You need to read the labels on the flour packages.

Now is the time to develop the good habit of asking bakeries, delicatessens and other places where you purchase prepared foods for the ingredients of foods you which to purchase. Tell the sales clerk that you have severe allergies and would like to buy their foods, but cannot unless you know the ingredients. Most places are very cooperative. If one of the ingredients is "flour," you need more information. Does the flour contain malt?

You will be able to find substitutes for most of these foods if you spend time looking for them. Just allow yourself extra time for the first two weeks; gradually, you will get to know what foods you can buy.

Vinegar is highly fermented. It is literally spoiled wine and is very concentrated in toxic yeast products. Vinegar is found in virtually all condiments, including ketchup and mustard, sauces and salad dressings.

Chocolate is the food that causes most people pause. You may be surprised to know that you can live without it. Chocolate has two problems. Chocolate is dried with a fungus. Chocolate also contains a chemical compound which is similar to one of the yeast chemicals. Unfortunately, there is no substitute for chocolate.

Pickles, pickled foods, soy sauce, worcestershire sauce and alcoholic beverages are fermented. Aged cheeses are highly mold contaminated. Cottonseed oil and cottonseed meal are problematic because the cottonseed plant is often mold contaminated and the products of the mold end up in the cottonseed oil.

Allowable Foods on Stage I-A

You can eat everything you now eat, except the specific foods eliminated (see the next page) This list gives you an overall idea. TIP: **For help in grocery shopping, see** *Shopping Lists* **(p. 95). Use all 3 lists.**

Fresh and freshly frozen Meat, Fish and Poultry: all kinds (preferably hormone and antibiotic free)
♦ Canned Tuna Fish (labelled "very low sodium"--only ingredients Tuna Fish and Water)
♦ Processed meats, including hot dogs, bacon, salami, luncheon meats and bologna

Fresh Produce: all kinds, including all fruits and vegetables, fresh and dried herbs

Dry Goods:
♦ Dried beans (all types)
♦ Coffee and tea
♦ Rice and all rice products
♦ Unprocessed clover honey
♦ Flour (malt free unbleached white flour, whole wheat, or gluten free flour made from other grains)
♦ Dried and packaged cereals without malt
♦ Chips that are not cooked in cottonseed oil or peanut oil
♦ Dried fruit and raisins
♦ Maple syrup
♦ Nuts and peanuts

♦ Oils-all except cottonseed and peanut
♦ Oatmeal and oats
♦ Pasta (whole wheat, semolina or rice)
♦ Sea salt
♦ Soda drinks
♦ Snack foods that are free of malt, chocolate and vinegar, including cookies, pretzels, and crackers
♦ Spices (cinnamon, etc.)
♦ Sugar
♦ Whole wheat tortillas or chapatis, matzah
♦ Whole wheat bread (malt free)
♦ Whole wheat flour

Milk, Butter and Eggs:
♦ Eggs, preferably hormone and antibiotic free
♦ Milk, all kinds
♦ Butter
♦ Cottage cheese, ricotta cheese, mozzarella and other non-aged cheeses
♦ Yogurt
♦ Ice Cream without chocolate or vanilla flavoring (try the new packaged sorbets!)
♦ Ice Cream substitutes (tofu or rice-based)

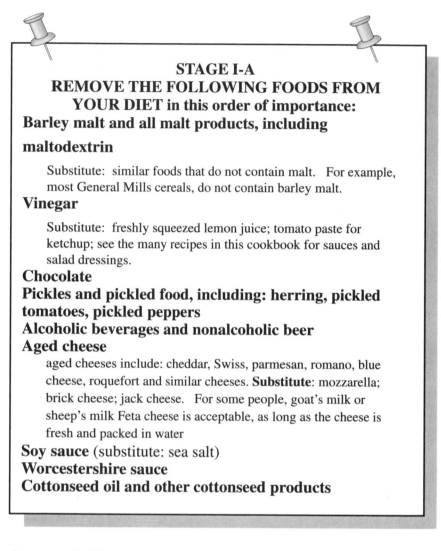

STAGE I-A
REMOVE THE FOLLOWING FOODS FROM
YOUR DIET in this order of importance:
Barley malt and all malt products, including
maltodextrin

> Substitute: similar foods that do not contain malt. For example, most General Mills cereals, do not contain barley malt.

Vinegar

> Substitute: freshly squeezed lemon juice; tomato paste for ketchup; see the many recipes in this cookbook for sauces and salad dressings.

Chocolate
Pickles and pickled food, including: herring, pickled tomatoes, pickled peppers
Alcoholic beverages and nonalcoholic beer
Aged cheese

> aged cheeses include: cheddar, Swiss, parmesan, romano, blue cheese, roquefort and similar cheeses. **Substitute**: mozzarella; brick cheese; jack cheese. For some people, goat's milk or sheep's milk Feta cheese is acceptable, as long as the cheese is fresh and packed in water

Soy sauce (substitute: sea salt)
Worcestershire sauce
Cottonseed oil and other cottonseed products

Stage I-B

On Stage I-B, you still can continue to use all of the recipes in this book except for the few containing apples. You also can use all of the foods on Shopping Lists 1, 2 and 3.

Stage I-B calls for removing more of the extremely fermented foods from your diet. The first food group to remove is nuts and peanuts, including all products made from nuts and peanuts (including peanut butter). Nuts and peanuts are inherently mold contaminated. Studies of peanut butter have shown large amounts of mold in peanut butter, the most mold being in natural (unprocessed) peanut butter. Many people also have peanut allergies.

The next food group covers apples and grapes and all products made from apples and grapes. Apples contain a natural antibiotic. Apples and grapes also contain yeast by-products that Dr. William Shaw, of the Great Plains Laboratory, has isolated. In clinical experience, apples, apple juice, grapes and grape juice wreak havoc in children sensitive to yeast. Substitute other fruits for apples and grapes. Pears substitute well for apples; fresh berries substitute well for grapes.

Coffee should be removed at this point. Coffee contains some of the same chemicals as malt. For some people, this may be the most difficult food to remove. Work at it slowly and gradually. I (Lori) know from personal experience how difficult giving up coffee may be. Substitute herbal tea and experiment with the wide variety of flavors you can find.

Finally, remove processed meats containing sodium nitrate and sodium nitrite. Sodium nitrite stabilizes the red color in processed meats and adds flavor. Sodium nitrate helps cure the meat and slowly breaks down into sodium nitrite. These additives have been linked to cancer. In my (Bruce) clinical experience, meats with these additives cause many children to have behavioral difficulties.

You should also add more good foods to your diet. By the time you start Stage I-B, brown rice should be a regular part of your diet. Concentrate now on increasing potatoes and vegetables, substituting other fruit for apples and grapes, such as plums, berries, and pears, and getting accustomed to drinking water instead of apple juice. We have delicious recipes for hot and cold lemonade in *Sweets & Treats*. The chapter called *Mainly Potatoes* will give you good ideas about how to use potatoes. Start experimenting, if you have not already done so, with different vegetable dishes from *Mainly Vegetables*. Almost all of the recipes in this book are suitable for Stage I-B.

Begin to add beans to your diet. Look at the chapter *Mainly Beans*, which will give you detailed cooking instructions for beans, as well as several delicious recipes. To introduce beans slowly, start cooking some of the many soups in this cookbook that use beans.   You will find that as you increase the amount of fiber in your diet, you will experience less gastric upset from beans. We also find that cooking beans in a slow cooker (directions in *Mainly Beans*) minimizes the amount of gas people get from eating beans.

Allowable Foods on Stage I-B

You can eat most things you now eat, except the specific foods eliminated from Stage I-A (p. 38) and now from Stage I-B (p. 41) This list gives you an overall idea.
TIP: For help in grocery shopping, see *Shopping Lists* (pages 95-98). Use all 3 lists.

Fresh and freshly frozen Meat, Fish and Poultry: all kinds (preferably hormone and antibiotic free)
♦ Canned Tuna Fish (labelled "very low sodium"--only ingredients Tuna Fish and Water)
♦ "Natural" hot dogs and luncheon meats only; nothing with sodium nitrates or sodium nitrites

Fresh Produce:
♦ All kinds except apples and apple products and grapes and grape products. These include all fruits and vegetables, fresh and dried herbs
♦ Fruit juices

Dry Goods:
♦ Dried beans (all types)
♦ Tea
♦ Rice and all rice products
♦ Unprocessed clover honey
♦ Flour (malt free unbleached white flour, whole wheat, or gluten free flour made from other grains)
♦ Dried and packaged cereals without malt
♦ Chips that are not cooked in cottonseed oil or peanut oil
♦ Dried fruit and raisins
♦ Maple syrup
♦ Oatmeal and oat products
♦ Oils-all except cottonseed, peanut, and other nut oils
♦ Pasta (whole wheat, semolina or rice)
♦ Sea salt

- Spices (cinnamon, etc.)
- Soda drinks
- Snack foods that are free of malt, chocolate and vinegar, including cookies, pretzels, and crackers
- Sugar
- Whole wheat tortillas or chapatis
- Whole wheat bread (malt free)
- Whole wheat flour

Milk, Butter and Eggs:
- Eggs, preferably hormone and antibiotic free
- Milk, all kinds
- Butter
- Cottage cheese, ricotta cheese, mozzarella and other non-aged cheeses
- Ice Cream without chocolate or vanilla flavoring (try the new packaged sorbets!)
- Ice Cream substitutes (tofu or rice-based)

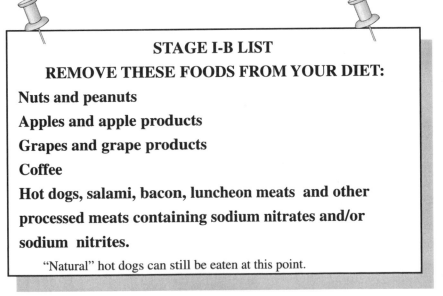

STAGE I-B LIST

REMOVE THESE FOODS FROM YOUR DIET:

Nuts and peanuts

Apples and apple products

Grapes and grape products

Coffee

Hot dogs, salami, bacon, luncheon meats and other processed meats containing sodium nitrates and/or sodium nitrites.

"Natural" hot dogs can still be eaten at this point.

Moving on: Stage II

Now that you are accustomed to Stage I, after a week to a few weeks, you should move on to Stage II if you still are not feeling 100 percent healthy, or if your health practitioner recommends moving on to Stage II. Some health care practitioners prefer to skip Stage II at this point and move directly to Stage III, eliminating wheat and milk, then going back to stage II. Skipping to Stage III particularly makes sense for health conditions such as autism.

For Stage II, make sure that you are eating brown rice instead of white rice, lots of good potatoes, beans and vegetables. Most of the recipes in *Feast Without Yeast* are suitable for Stage II. Use all of the foods on Shopping Lists 1 and 2, from the chapter called *Shopping Lists*.

You should follow Stage II for a period of four to six weeks, continuing with any other medical treatment , including taking nystatin. After consultation with your health care practitioner, you should consider moving on to Stage III.

The first foods to remove from your diet on Stage II are baked goods containing yeast, including bread. These foods actually contain yeast, and at this point, removing yeast will help. We give you several yeast free bread recipes in *Breads & Biscuits*.

Next, stop eating and cooking with corn and rye, which both are highly mold contaminated. Fermented foods to remove are: dried fruits and raisins, vanilla extract, concentrated fruit juice, and buttermilk.

Maple syrup should be removed. It contains some of the same toxic chemicals as vinegar, including acetol. Monosodium glutamate (MSG) and aspartame (brand name of NutraSweet) both are food additives that I have found, in my clinical experience, may cause headaches and other problems.

Stage II also calls for removing table sugar (sucrose) and substituting honey; not using colored spices, such as cinnamon, allspice, dried mustard, paprika, and so on, because many are inherently mold contaminated; mushrooms (a fungus); and carbonated sodas, most of which have corn based products in them, including carbonation.

I advise not using margarine at this point, too. Margarine has a host of problems. The human body does not metabolize it. Some studies have shown that the fats in margarine may be as bad for the body as highly saturated fats. Butter, a natural product, is much better for the body, even though it contains cholesterol. If you are trying to eliminate saturated fats or cholesterol, substitute oil for margarine (see *A Note on Ingredients* for a discussion about what type of oil to use).

Bananas are on the list because they are known to cause

migraines, and again, based on my clinical experience, cause problems for many people.

Spices, such as cinnamon, chili powder, cumin, dried mustard and all of the colored spices (not the green herbs) should be eliminated now. These spices cause problems for many people. They may be mold contaminated, or the processing may introduce harmful substances.

Finally, I advise cutting back on all meat and fish except veal and lamb, as I explained earlier. When yeast spoils meat, the toxic chemicals formed are worse than those formed by yeast in carbo- hydrate. In addition, chicken and pigs are fed cottonseed meal which is contaminated with a fungus called *Aspergillus*. I specu- late that the animals store the *Aspergillus* poisons in their fat. This technique is a common way for animals to handle poisons. It is possible that storing the fungus poisons is one reason why yeast sensitive patients should not eat large amounts of meat. See *Mainly Meats, Fish and Poultry* for easy to make recipes and cooking instructions.

Helpful foods for Stages I and II:
On Stage I, you added Brown Rice. Now, you only use Brown Rice.
At Stage II, increase:
Potatoes (all types)
Beans (all types)
Fresh Vegetables

See next page for the list of Allowable Foods for Stage II. . .

Allowable Foods on Stage II:

This list gives you an overall idea of which foods you can eat.   TIP: For help in grocery shopping, see *Shopping Lists*. Photocopy Lists 1, 2 and 3 and take them with you to the store.

Fresh and freshly frozen Meat, Fish and Poultry: all kinds (preferably hormone and antibiotic free). At this point, all types are permissible.
♦ Canned Tuna Fish (labelled "very low sodium"--only ingredients Tuna Fish and Water)
♦ "Natural" hot dogs and luncheon meats only; nothing with sodium nitrates or sodium nitrites

Fresh Produce:
♦ all kinds except apples and apple products, grapes and grape products, mushrooms and bananas. These include all fruits and vegetables, fresh and dried herbs

Dry Goods:
♦ Dried beans (all types)
♦ Tea
♦ Brown rice and all brown rice products
♦ Unprocessed clover honey
♦ Flour (malt free unbleached white flour, whole wheat flour and gluten free flour made from other grains, except rye and corn)
♦ Dried and packaged cereals without malt
♦ Potato chips that are not cooked in cottonseed, corn or peanut oil

♦ Oatmeal and oat products
♦ Oils: expeller pressed safflower oil, canola oil and olive oil
♦ Pasta (whole wheat, semolina or rice)
♦ Sea salt
♦ Snack foods and other processed foods that are free of: NutraSweet (aspartame); monosodium glutamate (MSG), malt, chocolate, yeast, vanilla extract, corn, rye and vinegar, including cookies, pretzels, matzah and crackers
♦ Whole wheat tortillas or chapatis
♦ Whole wheat flour (malt free)
♦ Yeast free bread from *Feast Without Yeast*

Milk, Butter and Eggs:
♦ Eggs, preferably hormone and antibiotic free
♦ Milk, all kinds except buttermilk
♦ Butter
♦ Yogurt
♦ Cottage cheese, ricotta cheese, mozzarella and other non-aged cheeses
♦ Ice Cream and Ice Cream substitutes without chocolate or vanilla flavoring

STAGE II

REMOVE THE FOLLOWING FOODS FROM YOUR DIET in this order of importance:

Baked goods containing yeast, including bread.

> Substitute: yeast free bread (***Delicious and Nutritious Whole Wheat Bread*** or other breads from ***Breads & Biscuits***), but <u>not</u> sourdough bread (sourdough is highly fermented).

Corn and rye

Vanilla extract

Dried fruits and raisins

Concentrated fruit juice, especially fruit juice concentrate used as a sweetener

Monosodium glutamate (MSG) and **Aspartame (NutraSweet)**

Maple syrup

Bananas

Meat and fish (cut back)

Spices

> These include colored spices, but not green herbs. (For example, cinnamon, cumin, dried mustard, chili powder, etc. Occasionally, spices may be OK.)

Mushrooms

Soda drinks and Buttermilk

Cooking oils except safflower oil, olive oil, and canola oil

> See *A Note on Ingredients.*

Table sugar (sucrose), including both white and brown.

> Substitute: unprocessed honey

Margarine

> Margarine has a host of problems. The human body does not metabolize it. Butter, a natural product, is much better for the body, even though it contains cholesterol. **Substitute: butter.**

Removing wheat/gluten and milk/casein: Stage III

This stage of the dietary changes takes you in a different direction. Because many people with yeast sensitivity also have gluten and casein sensitivity, I routinely advise patients who are still having problems to stop eating those foods.

What is gluten? Gluten (pronounced gloo'-ten) is a protein found in many grains, including wheat, rye, barley, oats, and some other grains. In the typical American diet, eliminating gluten means eliminating wheat. However, because so many other grains contain gluten, you will find that the main grain in your diet is rice. Corn is gluten free, but should not be eaten on a yeast free diet because corn is inherently mold contaminated. Other exotic gluten free grains include amaranth and quinoa. We do not use these grains and none of the recipes in *Feast Without Yeast* use them. If you choose to use exotic gluten free grains, you need to be sure that you are not sensitive to them. You also should purchase the grains from a source that refrigerates the grain, particularly after grinding into flour, to be sure that the grain is not mold contaminated.

What is casein? Casein (pronounced ka'-sene) is a protein found in milk and dairy products. On Stage III, you would eliminate all dairy products except butter. These include: milk, cottage cheese, yogurt, and so on. Follow Stage III for four to six weeks, continuing to consult with your health care practitioner.

Many recipes in this cookbook which are labelled "casein free" contain butter. Using butter on a milk/casein free diet is controversial. Butter is the fat from the milk, so it should not contain casein. However, in extreme cases of casein sensitivity, you should not use butter. Substitute safflower oil for the butter. If you have questions about whether you or your child can use butter safely, consult with your health care practitioner.

Why remove casein and gluten? Both milk and gluten contain substances that are toxic to the brains of sensitive people. When these substances are degraded by the body's digestive system, chemicals are released which resemble opioid chemicals. These chemicals are named opioids because they have effects on the brain similar to opiate drugs such as morphine, which affect pain systems. The brain has internal opioids which regulate the body's pain systems. The internal opioids are called endorphins. These food derived opioid chemicals are absorbed and react at receptors, or sites, for the body's own internal opioids.

The problem here is that opioids slow the brain down, so these chemicals hinder brain function. This is especially true for people with autism, and may likely be true for people suffering from Attention Deficit Disorder and other problems. In addition, yeast grow well in dilute milk so milk may aid yeast growth.

If you continue to feel that you need treatment, you probably are among the most severe in sensitivity. You then go on to Stage IV.

Very few patients go on to Stage IV--perhaps five to ten percent. That is only 5 or 10 people out of 100. However, we have designed *Feast Without Yeast* so it is safe and usable for everyone. Almost all of the recipes are suitable for people following Stage IV!

At this point, patients might consider testing or retesting their urine for yeast metabolites. See *Additional Resources* for further information. You also could consider testing for food allergies using immunological testing.

> **You will need to examine labels even more carefully at this point. Many foods contain hidden casein.** For example, many brands of soy cheese and rice cheese are labelled "dairy free" because they contain no lactose (a milk sugar that commonly causes problems), but they contain casein. Some brands of canned tuna fish contain casein. Look at each packaged food carefully.

Allowable Foods on Stage III:

This list gives you an overall idea of which foods you can eat.   TIP: For help in grocery shopping, see *Shopping Lists*. Photocopy Lists 1 and 2 and take them with you to the store.

Fresh and freshly frozen Meat, Fish and Poultry:
♦ all kinds (preferably hormone and antibiotic free). At this point, all types are permissible, but cut back on quantity.
♦ Canned Tuna Fish (labelled "very low sodium"--only ingredients Tuna Fish and Water)
♦ "Natural" hot dogs and luncheon meats only; nothing with sodium nitrates or sodium nitrites

Fresh Produce:
♦ all kinds except apples and apple products, grapes and grape products, mushrooms and bananas. These include all fruits and vegetables, fresh and dried herbs.

Dry Goods:
♦ Dried beans (all types)
♦ Tea
♦ Brown rice and all brown rice products

♦ Unprocessed clover honey
♦ Gluten free flour made from beans, rice or gluten free grains, such as amaranth and quinoa. No wheat, corn, rye, oat, barley flour.
♦ Rice cereals, such as puffed rice and cooked rice
♦ Potato chips that are not cooked in cottonseed, corn or peanut oil
♦ Oils: expeller pressed safflower oil, canola oil and olive oil
♦ Pasta (rice only)
♦ Sea salt
♦ Rice or potato based snack foods and other processed foods that are free of: wheat, milk, corn, rye, NutraSweet (aspartame); monosodium glutamate (MSG), malt, chocolate, yeast, vanilla extract, and vinegar

Butter and Eggs:
♦ Eggs, preferably hormone and antibiotic free
♦ Butter
♦ Ice Cream substitutes without chocolate or vanilla flavoring

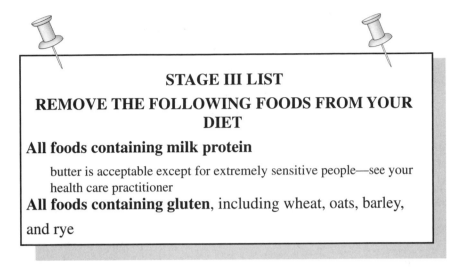

STAGE III LIST

REMOVE THE FOLLOWING FOODS FROM YOUR DIET

All foods containing milk protein

butter is acceptable except for extremely sensitive people—see your health care practitioner

All foods containing gluten, including wheat, oats, barley, and rye

The Final Step: Stage IV

Stage IV is the final stage of this process of dietary change. It appears to be restrictive, but in reality you still can enjoy a wide variety of tastes and textures. All of the foods on Shopping List 1 are fine. More than 80 percent of the recipes in *Feast Without Yeast* are suitable for Stage IV. Look for recipes that are designated "Suitable through Stage IV" in the gray box under the recipe title.

On a personal note, we have followed Stage IV for our son for several years. He is near the top of the growth charts in height and weight, and hardly ever gets sick.

Allowable Foods on Stage IV:
These are the foods you can eat.
TIP: For help in grocery shopping, see the chapter called *Shopping Lists*. Photocopy List 1 and take it with you to the store.

Fresh and freshly frozen Meat, Fish and Poultry:
♦ Veal and lamb are preferred. Occasionally, use hormone and antibiotic free chicken and turkey.

Fresh Produce:
♦ all fresh green vegetables except mushrooms
♦ lemons
♦ fresh and dried green herbs, such as basil, marjoram, dill, oregano, etc.
♦ raspberries
♦ blueberries
♦ blackberries
♦ cranberries
♦ boysenberries
♦ tomatoes
♦ potatoes
♦ sweet potatoes
♦ leeks, garlic, scallions and "spring onions"
♦ Mild chili peppers, such as Cubanel peppers
♦ Sweet (red) bell peppers

Dry Goods:
♦ Dried beans (all types)
♦ Brown rice and all brown rice products

♦ Unprocessed clover honey
♦ Gluten free flour made from beans or brown rice
♦ Rice cereals, such as puffed rice and cooked rice
♦ Oils: expeller pressed safflower oil, canola oil and olive oil
♦ Pasta (rice only)
♦ Sea salt
♦ Rice or potato based snack foods and other processed foods that are **free of:** wheat, milk, NutraSweet (aspartame); monosodium glutamate (MSG), malt, chocolate, yeast, vanilla extract, corn, rye and vinegar. Examine each piece carefully to be sure it has no green edges or other signs of mold contamination.

Butter and Eggs:
♦ Eggs, if tolerated. Many people who require Stage IV diets also are sensitive or allergic to eggs. If you can eat eggs, try to find hormone and antibiotic free eggs.
♦ Butter

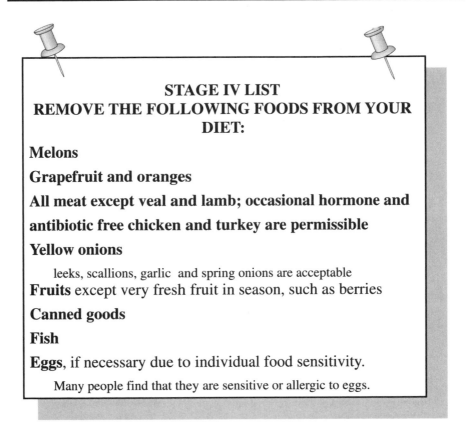

STAGE IV LIST
REMOVE THE FOLLOWING FOODS FROM YOUR DIET:

Melons

Grapefruit and oranges

All meat except veal and lamb; occasional hormone and antibiotic free chicken and turkey are permissible

Yellow onions

    leeks, scallions, garlic and spring onions are acceptable

Fruits except very fresh fruit in season, such as berries

Canned goods

Fish

Eggs, if necessary due to individual food sensitivity.

    Many people find that they are sensitive or allergic to eggs.

Now that you are living a yeast free life, you should feel much more comfortable. If you are not, you need to consult your health care practitioner to see if there are other problems hindering your health. If so, continue to use *Feast Without Yeast* as a guide to your everyday life. Use the recipes as a starting point for your cooking. Experiment with other allowable ingredients, and have fun!

On the following pages, you will find all of the lists in one place. . . .

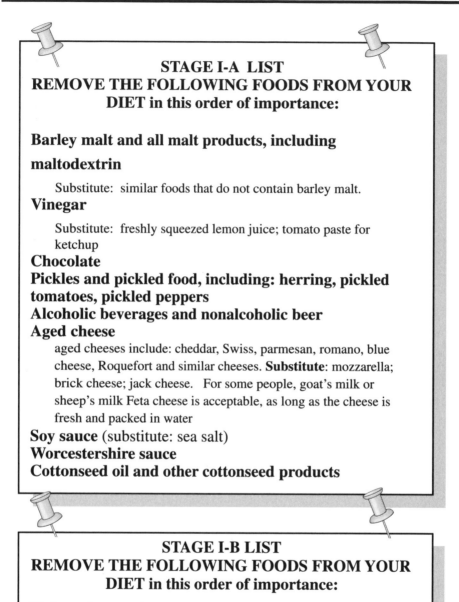

STAGE I-A LIST
REMOVE THE FOLLOWING FOODS FROM YOUR DIET in this order of importance:

Barley malt and all malt products, including maltodextrin

> Substitute: similar foods that do not contain barley malt.

Vinegar

> Substitute: freshly squeezed lemon juice; tomato paste for ketchup

Chocolate

Pickles and pickled food, including: herring, pickled tomatoes, pickled peppers

Alcoholic beverages and nonalcoholic beer

Aged cheese

> aged cheeses include: cheddar, Swiss, parmesan, romano, blue cheese, Roquefort and similar cheeses. **Substitute**: mozzarella; brick cheese; jack cheese. For some people, goat's milk or sheep's milk Feta cheese is acceptable, as long as the cheese is fresh and packed in water

Soy sauce (substitute: sea salt)

Worcestershire sauce

Cottonseed oil and other cottonseed products

STAGE I-B LIST
REMOVE THE FOLLOWING FOODS FROM YOUR DIET in this order of importance:

Nuts and peanuts

Apples and apple products

Grapes and grape products

Coffee

Hot dogs, salami, bacon, luncheon meats and other processed meats containing sodium nitrates and/or sodium nitrites.

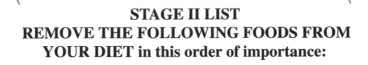

STAGE II LIST
REMOVE THE FOLLOWING FOODS FROM
YOUR DIET in this order of importance:

Baked goods containing yeast, including bread.

  Substitute: yeast free bread

Corn and rye

Vanilla extract

Dried fruits and raisins

Concentrated fruit juice, especially fruit juice

concentrate used as a sweetener

Monosodium glutamate (MSG) and **Aspartame**

(NutraSweet)

Maple syrup

Bananas

Meat and fish (cut back)

Spices

  (Cinnamon, cumin, chili powder, etc. Colored spices, but not
  green herbs.)

Mushrooms

Soda drinks and Buttermilk

Cooking oils except safflower oil, olive oil, and canola

oil

  See *A Note on Ingredients.*

Table sugar (sucrose), including both white and brown.

  Substitute: unprocessed honey

Margarine

  margarine has a host of problems. The human body does not
  metabolize it. Butter, a natural product, is much better for the
  body, even though it contains cholesterol. **Substitute: butter**

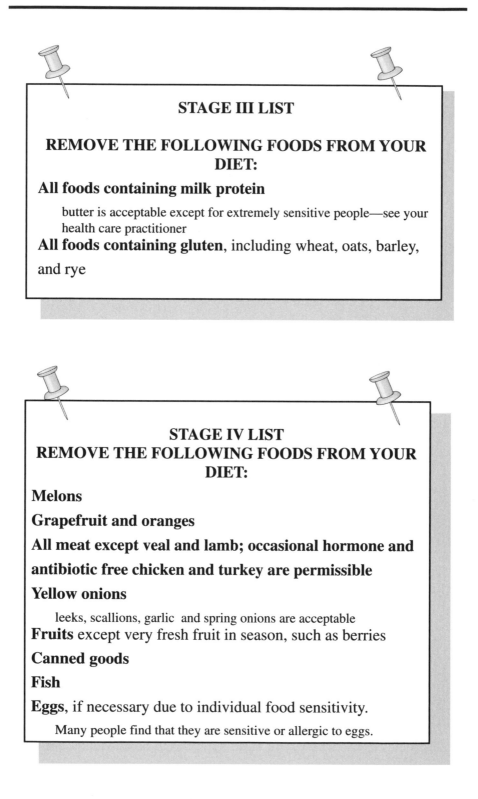

STAGE III LIST

REMOVE THE FOLLOWING FOODS FROM YOUR DIET:

All foods containing milk protein

> butter is acceptable except for extremely sensitive people—see your health care practitioner

All foods containing gluten, including wheat, oats, barley, and rye

---

STAGE IV LIST
REMOVE THE FOLLOWING FOODS FROM YOUR DIET:

Melons

Grapefruit and oranges

All meat except veal and lamb; occasional hormone and antibiotic free chicken and turkey are permissible

Yellow onions

> leeks, scallions, garlic and spring onions are acceptable

Fruits except very fresh fruit in season, such as berries

Canned goods

Fish

Eggs, if necessary due to individual food sensitivity.

> Many people find that they are sensitive or allergic to eggs.

The Four Stages for Children

*Children present special challenges for implementing dietary change. This chapter covers what those challenges are, as well as basic techniques for changing your child's diet to improve his or her health. We also give you a list of substitutions you can make to transition your child to eating different foods, and recipes that we know from experience kids love to eat. We do not repeat information from the previous chapter, **The Four Stages**, so be sure you read both before attempting to change your child's diet.*

C hildren may have many of the conditions which a yeast free, and possibly wheat and milk free diet can help. These conditions range from autism and attention deficit disorder, to eczema. Yet children are among my toughest patients because they have little direct control over their food when young, and too much control when older! Implementing the four stages with and for children is not so difficult if you approach the task as a process. Go slowly and gently, and use lots of substitutions at first, even if you know the foods you use as substitutes may be eliminated later. This chapter will give you a road map to follow for children.

The subject of food and children has been debated and argued extensively. Each culture and generation seems to view differently the amount of control a parent should have over a child's food. Certainly, you cannot control what a child actually eats by forcing the child to eat, any more than you can control when a child needs to use the bathroom. However, you can control what choices are available to a child, even in social settings.

> Key Thought #1: Change the way you think about food from sustenance or pleasure to health and safety.

The first overall key to success in implementing the four stages with children is to change the way you—and consequently your children—think about food. Food is no longer just an issue of basic sustenance or pleasure. It is a health and safety issue. For example, if you found out that your child was diabetic and might go into a coma if you allowed the child to eat certain foods, you would do your best to keep your child away from those foods. Accidents may happen, but you would try to minimize those accidents.

Likewise, the conditions from which children suffer, with which this diet can help, are threatening to their health and safety. You, as a parent, need to move "food" issues surrounding their health issues into the same category that you would view medication issues. Do you give your child the choice of whether or not to take medication for diabetes? If not, move this diet into the same category. If you give your child those types of choices, then treat this diet in the same manner.

You, as a parent, should begin observing and becoming aware of the connection between your child's eating problematic foods and their uncomfortable health consequences. In your child, bad foods may cause headaches, diarrhea, constipation, itching, screaming, or other unpleasant side effects. These health consequences may occur anywhere from a few minutes to a few days later, depending on the sensitivity of the child.

Without a guidebook like *Feast Without Yeast*, becoming aware of food's unpleasant side effects requires an incredible amount of detective work and a completely open mind. We write this based on our own experience. In hindsight, it is easy for us to see which foods cause our son's problems. Milk, wheat and eggs cause itching and eczema. Melons cause headaches. Chocolate causes migraines. The list goes on and on. However, when he was younger, the relationship was not so clear.

I recall taking our son to a "Mommy and Me" recreation class when he was four. He would do great until snack time, eat snack, and his behavior would become totally unmanageable. He became uncooperative; he cried; he refused to participate in activities he enjoyed. People offered various explanations: breaking his rhythm and introducing another activity caused him to lose focus; he was tired, and so on. In reality, the class made creative snacks, using ingredients such as peanut butter, dried milk and coconut— all ingredients we now know are highly toxic to him.

For another example, our son also used to be relatively calm before bed, then we'd give him a bedtime snack of a natural cereal and milk. Then, zoom! Off he'd be flying like a rocket. Two or three frustrating hours later, he'd be asleep. One friend who observed this behavior suggested maybe the snack had something to do with it, but we (unfortunately) shrugged off this suggestion. Years later, we found out that our son was allergic or sensitive to the milk and most of the ingredients in the cereal, including malted barley flour. Bedtime is a lot easier now.

Even for people aware that food can have an effect on behavior and health, discovering these links, without help, can be difficult. We wrote this book so you would not have to go through those same struggles!

You need not be totally aware of all of the connections between food and health in order to start treating your child. Over time, as you implement the Four Stages, you will become much more aware of the connection between ingesting certain foods and unhealthy consequences. After a few weeks on Stage I, your child may experience, perhaps for the first time in her life, physical comfort and well being. The healthy consequences of eating good foods, and the unhealthy consequences of eating foods that are bad for her, will become more obvious to you and to her. As you notice these consequences and connect them with your child getting into something bad for her, you can discuss with your child that eating that food, is causing her headache, or itching, or lack of attention, or whatever it is. Your child will then begin to associate certain foods with physical feelings and learn to make good choices on her own. We personally have experienced this and have observed this in our own children and in others.

Key Thought #2: Even though you are in a hurry to help your child, slow down. Make the transition gradual.

After you have begun to treat food as a health and safety issue, the second overall key to implementing this diet, ironically, is to go slowly. Be patient with yourself and your child and treat the inevitable mistakes as learning experiences. You are making dramatic changes for the long run, not just experimenting with a short term "diet." Mistakes and poor choices will happen. You will inadvertently offer your child something he or she shouldn't have, and will see bad consequences. Your child will trade foods with someone at school. This is part of life. In fact, much of our experience is based on what I call trial and error—mostly error!

When we first began eliminating foods, we made many mistakes and saw their consequences very clearly. Although we regret that our child had to suffer due to our mistakes, those mistakes crystallized for us and for those around us the connections between eating certain foods and having certain health problems. We hope that you do not make as many mistakes.

As you begin to understand that there are ways in which your child can feel better and your household can run more smoothly, when the bad times come, you will not feel so desperate and hopeless. We have had many sleepless nights, headaches, and other problems caused by eating the wrong foods. We know that these times are terrible for our son and for the family, but we always reflect back on how life was before we intervened at all in our son's food choices. The screaming was constant; the itching was intolerable. So a few days will pass, then he is on the right track again.

Typically, we find that bad foods take about three days to move completely through a sensitive child's system. So, bear with the problems for those days, give your child something to ease the symptoms, whether it be ibuprofen or something for itching, or whatever helps, and know that the problem will go away. If after three days the problem does not ease up, *be sure to see your health care practitioner.* **IF YOU SEE EXTREME OR LIFE THREATENING CONDITIONS, DO NOT WAIT THREE DAYS. SEE YOUR HEALTH PROFESSIONAL IMMEDIATELY.**

Now that you see food as a health and safety issue and are prepared for a gradual, less than perfect transition, you can begin to implement the diet pragmatically. We suggest following the nine pointers for success we give in the rest of the chapter.

1 ▶ Teach your child that food is a health and safety issue, not just a matter of taste.

Teach your child what you are learning: food is a health and safety issue. This step may seem obvious, but it bears remembering that you are training your child for eventual independence in a world full of food choices that may not be good for her. You can begin teaching, even at three or four years old, that certain foods make them feel bad and others help them feel good. Teach your children that avoiding foods is not deprivation—it is giving them the help they need and deserve to live a good life.

Use both positive and negative reinforcement in your teaching. This is called behavior modification, and is something most parents do without thinking. Positive reinforcement includes anything that motivates your child (except, of course, bad foods). Reward your child with praise or other motivating item, for eating the right foods and also for avoiding the foods that are bad choices for him. While using positive reinforcement for doing the right thing, use negative reinforcement to remind the child that the food he avoided would have caused a headache, or inattention, or whatever the effect is. Remember that no child likes to be in pain or feel out of control.

Negative reinforcement does not mean punishment in the traditional sense. Negative reinforcement in this context is more effective if you emphasize cause and effect. Do not punish your child for eating the wrong foods. Your child's punishment is feeling bad. Rather, tell him "you got a headache/became hyper/ [whatever] because you ate [chocolate/cheese/whatever the offending food is]." Patiently teaching cause and effect will pay off in the long run. Your child will learn to avoid foods without parental intervention, because he will know that eating certain foods causes him to feel bad.

In summary, you must teach your child that food is a health and safety issue by using both positive and negative reinforcement. Find out what motivates your child and use that motivation to help your child become independent and healthy!

> 2 ▶ Provide healthy, great tasting food for your child.

Give your child great tasting food. Being healthy does not mean living a life without the pleasures that we associate with food. Many parents avoid changing diet because they are afraid to take away foods their child appears to enjoy eating. How can they take away their child's one pleasure? We have had this experience and can tell you that once you substitute good foods for the foods that bother your child, your child's quality of life will improve. Food will no longer be your child's only source of pleasure.

Our son's favorite meal used to be tofu dogs topped with ketchup, mustard, salsa and mayonnaise, accompanied by popcorn topped with ketchup. This was at a time when he was screaming most of the time; food seemed to be his main pleasure in life. Now we know he cannot eat soy (tofu); he gets migraines from the vinegar in ketchup, mustard, salsa and mayonnaise, and he is allergic to corn. We had to exercise parental judgment to take away those favorite foods, but he became much happier because the headaches went away. Food was no longer his only source of pleasure in life. We have seen this happen with other children as well, even with the pickiest eaters.

While the above example may be extreme, due to our son's extreme sensitivity, we know how difficult these parental choices are. We urge you to make them in your child's best interests. In my experience as a doctor, I have found that when parents begin substituting nutritionally good and great tasting food for foods that cause problems, the children begin to feel better and eventually want to eat the better food. This even happens with the children who are viewed as the pickiest eaters, because they no longer fear that everything they try will hurt their stomachs.

The change in foods may be as subtle as substituting good oil (safflower) for bad oil. One child we know to be a very picky eater happily devoured our **Crispy Potato Latkes**, made only with potatoes, salt and safflower oil, when he wouldn't eat similar food at home. The only difference was the oil.

What follows are suggestions first, for direct substitutions (food for food), and second, for recipes from this book that you can use to tempt your child to eat better foods overall. Initially, you will need to look at your cupboards and determine which foods contain vinegar and/or malt. Then you can go shopping for other brands that do not contain the offending substances. You will be surprised at how many you can find.

<u>Old Food:</u>	<u>New Food:</u>
Ketchup	Tomato paste (thinned)
Hot chocolate	**Hot Spicy Milk** (p.362) **Hot Lemonade** (p.364)
Fast food french fries	**French Fries Just Like in the Restaurants, but Better** (p.248)
Bread baked with yeast	**Delicious and Nutritious Whole Wheat Bread** (p.182) Rice Cakes (commercial, made only with brown rice and salt; no flavored rice cakes)
Table sugar	Unprocessed honey
Vinegar	Freshly squeezed lemon juice
Maple syrup	Unprocessed honey
Soy sauce or Tamari	Sea salt
Products containing Malt	Similar products without malt

More often than not, you will substitute great foods kids love to eat for foods you have eliminated. Here are just some of the recipes you can try out to start:

Recipes Kids Love:

Breads & Biscuits:

Light 'N Flaky Whole Wheat Biscuits (p.192)
Delicious and Nutritious Whole Wheat Bread (p.182)
Light and Fluffy Pancakes and Variations (p.194)
Pizza Bread (p.190)

Mainly Potatoes:

Hash Browns (p.252)
French Fries Just Like in the Restaurants (p.248)
Quick & Easy French Fries (p.250)
Mashed Potatoes (p.251)
Dilled Potatoes (p.245)
Crispy Traditional Potato Latkes (p.255)
Crispy Potato Latkes Without Wheat or Eggs (p.256)

Mainly Beans:

Hot Beans (p.201)
Five Minute Special Stir-Fried Beans (p.204)
Tomato Beans (p.208)
Herbed Zucchini Lentils (p.218)
Lentils, Plain and Simple (p.206)
Vegetarian Baked Beans (p.210)
Thick and Meaty Bean Burgers (p.214)
Lean and Tasty Bean Burgers (p.211)
Lemon Garbanzo Beans (p.201)
Whole Wheat Burritos (p.217)

More on the next pages. . . . .

Dressings and Sauces:

Creamy Cucumber Dressing (p.101)
Fresh Basil and Tomato Sauce (p.105)
Fresh Pizza Tomato Sauce (p.107)
Quick 'N Easy Tomato Sauce (p.110)
Tomato, Dill and Marjoram Sauce (p.111)
Hummus (p.121)
Pear Sauce (p.120)

Mainly Rice:

Basic Brown Rice (p. 232)
Fluffy Rice (p.237)
Vegetable Fried Rice (p.220)
Zucchini Tomato Fried Rice (p.224)
Rice Burgers (p.235)
Rice-Ta-Touille (p.228)
Tomato Rice (p.230)
Sticky Rice (p.236)
Thanksgiving Stuffing (p.240)

Sweets & Treats:

Hot Lemonade (p.364)
Fresh Cold Lemonade (p.363)
Hot Spicy Milk (p.362)
Rolled Butter Cookies (p.324)
Everyone's Favorite Oatmeal Cookies (p.323)
Valentine's Day Cookies (p.325)
The Best Carrot Cake in the Whole World (p.312)
Pumpkin Cake (p.315)
Fruit Pie (p.336)
Blueberry Pie Filling (p.337)
Baked Crustless Blueberry Pie (p.339)
Honey Butter Cream Frosting (p.341)
Fun and Flavorful Butter Cream Frosting (p.342)
All the sorbets and ice milks (pp.350-362)

Mainly Meat, Fish and Poultry:

Spaghetti Sauce with Meatballs (p.302)
Roasted Chicken with Herbs (p.297)
Veal Stew (p.298)
Veal Meatballs and Potatoes (p.307)
Basic Tuna Salad (p.296)
Garden Lasagna with Meat (p.304)

Spectacular Soups:

Cream of Pizza Soup (p.161)
Thick 'N Chunky Tomato Soup (p.148)
Cream of Zucchini Soup (p.158)
Cream of Broccoli Soup (p.159)
Cream of Broccoli and Zucchini Soup (p.160)
Creamy Harvest Soup (p.163)
Birthday Minestrone (pp.138-39)
Vegetable Soup for Matzah Balls (p.145)
Vegetarian Matzah Balls (p.144)
Rice & Dill Dumplings (p.146)
Italian Vegetable Soup (p.149)
Zucchini Lentil Soup (p.154)

Mainly Vegetables:

Stir Fried Zucchini with Tomatoes P.262)
Zucchini Surprise (p.269)
Stir Fried Chinese Cabbage or Bok Choy (p.273)
Carrot Tzimmes (p.278)
Garden Lasagna (p.280)
Roasted Pumpkin Seeds (p.283)

Birthday Cakes:

For Stages I & II, use *The Best Carrot Cake in the Whole World* (p. 312) or *Pumpkin Cake* (p.315) with *Honey Buttercream Frosting* (p.341) or *Fun and Flavorful Frosting* (p. 342)

For Stages III & IV, use *Birthday Sorbet Cake* (p.358) with *Honey Butter Frosting* (p.343)

3 Enlist the support of other people who have contact with your child.

Enlist the support of other people who have contact with your child. These people include teachers, other relatives, therapists and friends. Teach them not only which foods are not allowed, but also which are allowed. Explain to them the health reasons behind the restrictions, but also explain to them that your child feels better and suffers less by working within the dietary guidelines than by having lots of food available to her that makes her feel bad. If your child is in special education, place the list of foods to be avoided in his or her Individual Education Plan. For all children, make sure that you send a letter to school for the principal, teachers and support staff, explaining the food restrictions. Schools will honor these restrictions. Remember, if somebody does not know about the food restrictions, they cannot ensure your child's safety. Mistakes may happen, but ideally they will happen less often if the list is provided in writing.

4 Always be prepared for temptation--have good food choices available for your child.

Always be prepared for temptation. Your child will encounter many situations in life where she will be tempted to eat the wrong foods. Make sure your child has good food available at all times. When traveling, pack picnics for your child to eat in the car, on planes, busses and trains. You may be able to serve your child some purchased food, but usually you won't know beforehand whether this is an option. At some restaurants, you can get baked potatoes, salad with lemon, or plain rice. Order special meals on airplanes. We have found that the diabetic meals and fruit plates are the safest choices. Experiment with your airline's special meals.

Send your child's food to school, including snacks and lunch. Assume that institutional food is filled with things that will affect your child's health, unless you find out otherwise. Usually, you can keep some safe foods at the school for snack time to be served with the other children's snacks. In some schools, social life revolves around "hot lunch." If this is the case in your school, discuss with the teachers ways to decrease the social emphasis on hot lunch, and increase the importance of socializing during lunch time, no matter who prepares the lunch.

Carry snacks around for small children. You can share your snacks with your child's friends, if their parents approve. Children often like to eat what everyone else is eating, and will enjoy sharing their food.

5 Make your child's health a family priority, and get the entire family involved in eating different foods.

Make your child's health a family priority. This sounds odd— of course, your child's health is a family priority! What we mean is that at least for the first few weeks while attempting to implement dietary change, your entire family should follow the four stages during community meals. We say this for a few reasons. First, children should feel safe at home. You can keep food that is unacceptable for your child, but OK for other children in the family, in a locked cupboard to be eaten out of the affected child's presence. As your child grows older and more aware of the problems that foods can cause him, he will be able to tolerate having forbidden food around the house. Second, the other family members will learn that changing diet is not so bad, and will be less tempted to feel sorry for your child or feed him foods that cause bad reactions on the sly to help him feel better.

6   Ally yourself with sympathetic health care professionals.

Ally yourself with sympathetic health care professionals, who will help you in your quest to help your child, without undermining your attempts. Again, this sounds odd. Why would a health care practitioner undermine a parent's desire to help his or her child? Our experience, as parents and as professionals, is that most health professionals and other health care practitioners care very much about their patients. They will not undermine parental efforts maliciously or even consciously, recognizing that parents know their children best and are motivated to help them. Health care professionals are rightly suspicious of fads and trends that later prove to be worthless or even harmful.

Occasionally, however, parents will attempt the harmless intervention of dietary change, and some health care professionals will undermine these attempts to help the child by not listening, by lack of support, or by other more intrusive means.

Our suggestion is that you discuss with your health professionals what you are thinking about doing, or what you are doing, and give them the benefit of your personal observations about your own child. See whether your health professional is willing to listen to you about what you observe. Nobody has anything to gain from your personal experience except you and your family.

Many physicians, in particular, have been taught and truly believe that there is no relationship between the food that someone eats and that person's health. Many health care professionals undermine parental effort simply by refusing to believe parental observation that their child improved due to a change in diet. (This pattern of disbelief does not appear to be as true between health professionals and adult patients.)

One recent example reported to us involves an infant in a family we know very well. The child, just over a year old, began to vomit three to four times a day and to develop asthma. Fortunately, the child's pediatrician recommended eliminating milk from the child's diet to see what happened before doing invasive tests and putting the child on steroids for the asthma. Within one day, the child was better. Within a few months, the child had no symptoms at all of stomach distress or asthma. The pediatrician was convinced that removing the milk was effective. However, another doctor, a specialist, could not or would not believe that removing milk would have that effect. He still recommended going through the tests and the medications for asthma. I suspect that had this child had the same miraculous cure after going on a medication, that specialist would have lauded the curative powers of medication. (The parents did not follow the specialist's advice!)

Do we indict all doctors? Certainly not! I (Bruce) am a doctor, as are the individuals who pioneered observations about the connections between yeast and poor health, such as Dr. William Crook and Dr. Orian Truss. Many pediatricians and other physicians support the idea that food is connected to health. The point is this: some doctors and health care professionals believe that food and health are related, and some don't. This is similar to many other debates within medicine, including whether asthma is related to allergies, whether to use antibiotics immediately to treat every ear infection or whether to wait, how to handle childbirth issues, and so on.

You as a parent should find out what your health care professional's bias is about food and health. If that person has a bias against nutritional intervention, but is a great health professional in all other respects, you can make an informed choice about whether you are willing to pursue nutritional intervention despite your health professional's lack of support. If you are not willing to do so, change health professionals. There are many excellent health professionals out there.

We have been fortunate in finding physicians who listen to us, support our choices for our child, and offer advice, as long as they see that what we do for our child does not harm him and does, in fact, help him. Before finding these health professionals, we have had a difficult time confronting the bias against dietary intervention in some physicians we have encountered. The first allergist to whom we took our son assured us that none of our son's problems could be related to allergies because he did not have a runny nose. He refused to do further testing, even though our son suffered tremendous skin problems. We learned later that he had a very narrow view of allergies, even among allergists. We could not get pain medication from our pediatrician for our son's migraines because the evidence of migraines was based solely on our clinical observations, not on emergency room visits and procedures.

In my clinical experience, many, many parents are dissuaded from trying dietary change to help their children due to their physician's lack of support. Patients come to see me for help, start changing diet, notice immediate effects, then go back to their pediatricians, who often say, "No, changing diet could not possibly have had this effect. Your child just spontaneously got better." Many of these patients then stop the dietary changes because they are afraid to cross their health professionals. The children lose their gains and end up on a treadmill of medications.

When choosing a health professional, question the health professional about his or her views on diet and health. Even if your health professional does not prescribe this treatment, you want him or her to listen to what you are doing and to support your efforts to help your child, not to undermine them.

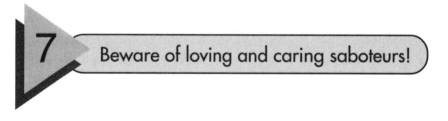

7   Beware of loving and caring saboteurs!

Even following all of these guidelines, you may run into problems. Unfortunately, sabotage, in the guise of feeling sorry for a child, is common. The sabotage may be subtle or overt, and may come from strangers or even other loving and doting family members. This idea is abhorrent to many, and they have not hesitated to criticize us for raising it. However, I have seen enough instances of what I call loving sabotage to bring it to your attention.

Some people around your child may never want to accept the fact that you are helping your child by changing his diet. These people may slip your child chocolate or soda, because these people are so used to the idea that food is a tremendous source of pleasure, and cannot cause pain. They truly believe that what you are doing is depriving your child of pleasure—therefore causing pain—and may not want to see how much better your child feels. Therefore, in their minds, they are helping the child by offering treats. Unfortunately, these people are almost never around when the bad effects set in, or if they are, don't believe that the effects are from food.

This sabotage can occur even in a totally controlled setting. I (Bruce) had a patient in an institution who initially did very well on Stage I of the diet. She began declining for unknown reasons. At a staffing, it came out that an aide felt sorry for this patient and was giving her M&M's!

At the same institution, a young man was doing well on the diet, but later stopped eating. It turned out that a staff member had told theyoung man that if he stopped eating, they'd take him off of this " crazy diet".

We suggest that if your child is having attacks of problems you thought you had eliminated, gently, but closely, question all of the people who have contact with your child to find out exactly what the child may have eaten.

> **8** Gently educate your friends and relatives that you are working with your child's diet to help your child, not to change <u>their</u> life-styles.

A second problem you may encounter is the loving relative or friend who perceives your approach to your child's problem as an attack on their manner of living or child rearing. This becomes a problem for you and your child because, in my (Bruce) experience, any ensuing discussions become arguments which in turn tend to become highly personalized and divorced from the issue of whether your child's health is improving.

Your child may see and hear this dissension and believe that he or she caused it.

This problem is unfortunate. The best way to avoid it is to try to explain that you are attempting to help your child be an independent, healthy person. You are not attacking their life-style or food choices. What is good for your friend or relative may not be good for your child. These people need to understand that food affects your child's health much the same as food affects a diabetic or a heart patient's health. Give these people a copy of this cookbook so they can read what you have read and can make great tasting food for your child!

9 Examine everything that enters your child's digestive system, including medications, vitamins and nonfood items.

Even if you are doing everything right, your child still may be having problems that you and your health practitioner cannot solve. If this is the case, you need to recheck everything that goes into your child's mouth, including medications, vitamins and nonfoods. Medications and vitamins, especially childrens' preparations, often contain substances that extremely sensitive children cannot tolerate. These substances include artificial colors and flavors, and/or artificial sweeteners such as aspartame (NutraSweet). Liquid preparations often contain alcohol.

One of our early experiences taught us this lesson. We would give our son children's acetaminophen (for example, brand name of Tylenol) to help his headaches. The medicine seemed to make the headaches worse. This medicine turned out to contain aspartame as well as artificial colors, flavors and fillers.

The best way to solve this problem is to have your health professional prescribe any medication in the pure, or "compounded", form. Most major metropolitan areas have at least one pharmacy that is a compounding pharmacy. The pharmacy will give you the pure medication, which you then can mix in something the child does not mind eating, such as unprocessed honey.

Beware that most medications naturally taste like poison, which is why pharmaceutical companies dress them up in all of the flavorings to begin with!

In addition, when you are taking your child's food intake survey, check to make sure your child is not ingesting any non-foods. A very small percentage of people find soap, plants, wood, dirt and other nonfood items particularly appealing.

Some children eat these foods overtly. Other children are more subtle. They may rub plant leaves and taste the juices, or play in dirt, then lick their fingers, or suck on their fingernails to get at soap that may be trapped beneath.

In the medical literature, this is called "PICA." You may have to follow your child around for a day or two to observe what is going on.

Many people believe these non-foods are relatively harmless, but they are not. Be vigilant about eliminating these non-foods, too. In addition to the physical harm that eating non-foods can cause (perforated intestines is one), the toxins inherent in these items, as well as added toxins (mold on plants, furniture polish, and so on) are extremely dangerous to a sensitive child.

We have seen extreme behavioral changes due to ingestion of soap and plants, in particular, including anxiety, aggression, depression, and lack of cooperation with other therapies. These behavioral changes dissipate as the offending toxin moves out of the child's body. This process usually takes about three days.

Having a child or children with extreme sensitivities to yeast, mold, fermentation, and often milk, wheat and eggs, is extremely difficult and requires considerable patience on the part of parents and everyone around the child. The results are worth the effort in the end, though. You will have a happier, healthier child.

Notes for Parents of Picky Eaters:

One of the most common parental concerns is whether a "picky eater" will survive the Four Stages.

The answer is "yes."

As we have explained above, one reason children become picky eaters is that foods disagree with them. They find the foods that make them feel good, and fear other foods. Ironically, however, the foods that make children feel good may make them feel worse in the long run. Children don't know this. As parents, you need to recognize that even if your child truly loves a certain food, your child should not eat that food if the food is bad for him or her.

Once you begin to substitute foods that taste great <u>and</u> do not hurt your child, your child will begin to enjoy eating a greater repertoire of foods. This takes time.

We advise parents to follow three hard and fast rules relating to their picky eaters:

Never comment on your child's picky eating to anyone within earshot of your child. Better yet, never comment on it at all. We cannot tell you how many times we have offered children new foods that they might just love, the child appears interested, then the well intentioned parent says, "oh, Johnny will never eat that." Of course, Johnny takes the cue from Mom or Dad and refuses the new food. A matching principle is to **always model good eating behavior**. As you eat the foods you want your child to eat, say things like, "this is really delicious. I'm glad I'm eating it."

Always praise your child for eating anything good, double the praise for trying new foods, and don't push too hard. A child may only be comfortable trying one food or one bite at a time.

Give your child credit for being smart. When most children begin to connect feeling good with eating good foods, they want to eliminate the bad foods and eat the good foods. One of our young friends (age 9) started Stage I-A. After a few days felt so much better he voluntarily gave up chocolate!

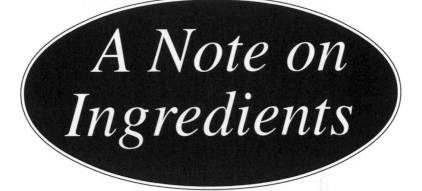

A Note on Ingredients

In this chapter, we go through some of the specific ingredients that we use throughout this cookbook and explain

~ *Why we use certain ingredients*

~ *How to prepare them*

~ *Some alternative ingredients*

Beans

All recipes use dried beans unless otherwise noted. For complete instructions on using beans, see the chapter called **Mainly Beans** in this cookbook.

Barley

The recipes using barley call for "hulled" barley. Hulled barley is the barley version of brown rice. The tough, inedible outer hull has been removed, but the thin layer of brown fiber, vitamins and minerals surrounding the barley kernel remains. The usual type of barley, "pearled" barley, lacks this layer of fiber, vitamins and minerals, just as white rice lacks the fiber, vitamins and minerals of brown rice.

Because barley contains gluten, brown rice may be substituted for gluten free versions of barley recipes, where noted. The rice version will not be as thick as the barley version.

Cooking Spray

Occasionally, you may want to use nonstick cooking spray to grease pans. Be sure you use cooking spray that is acceptable for your stage of the diet. Canola oil or Safflower oil cooking spray is acceptable for Stage IV. Many cooking oils contain corn or soy.

Fruit- Fresh and Frozen

Some of the recipes, particularly sorbets, use fresh or freshly frozen fruit. Good rules of thumb are: avoid packaged fruit; use only fruit in season (not exotic fruits out of season), and make sure the fruit is firm and ripe, but not soft and overripe. After purchasing fruit, check the fruit carefully for mold or rot and, where possible, cut out the bad spots. Throw out or compost bad fruit.

We make it a practice to purchase fresh raspberries, blueberries and blackberries in season, either directly from growers or from good produce markets, and freeze the berries.   That way, we have an ample supply of fresh, frozen berries to use all year. Sometimes we make a fun day out of storing winter berries by going to "pick it yourself" places.

Berries can be frozen by spreading the berries out on a cookie sheet, placing in the freezer for 12-24 hours, the storing in reusable plastic freezer bags. Date the bags and use within a year.

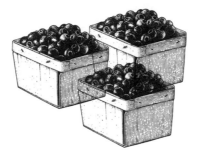

Herbs and Spices

Green herbs are fine. Generally, people on a yeast free diet do not tolerate the spices as well. Green herbs include such things as basil, dill, oregano, marjoram, thyme, and so on. Dill seeds, celery seeds also are fine. Spices include such things as cumin, curry powder, mustard, coriander, cardamom, cinnamon, allspice, cloves, and so on. Occasionally, we use spices such as cinnamon, allspice and cloves. Used only occasionally, these seem to be OK through Stage I. We eliminate spices at Stage II. Judge based on your own experience with these spices. **If you are sensitive to these spices, PLEASE DO NOT USE THEM.**

All recipes call for dried herbs, unless the recipe specifically states "fresh" herbs. If you wish to use fresh herbs, use three times the amount as for dried herbs (for example, instead of 1 tsp. dried basil, you would use 1 T. [3 tsp.] fresh, chopped basil).

Honey

We recommend only fresh, unprocessed honey. Processed honey has been heated and has fewer nutrients available than unprocessed honey. We prefer the taste of clover honey, which is the lightest and sweetest tasting honey, so most recipes call for clover honey. However, there are more than 200 flavors of honey!

Please experiment with other flavors to see which ones you like best. Some honeys are very strong (buckwheat, for example), others more tart (cranberry). The taste of your recipe will change according to the type of honey you use.

For the best fresh honey, check your local farmers' markets. Ask when the honey was processed and whether the grower heated the honey before putting the honey in jars. Purchase only the current season's honey and purchase natural, unprocessed honey. You usually can purchase enough in the fall to last all winter. We have found that local growers often do not mind making midwinter deliveries, if you purchase honey in sufficient quantity.

As a rule of thumb, our family of five goes through about one gallon (12 pounds) of honey every 6-8 weeks, and we do very little baking!

Lemon Juice

Many recipes use lemon juice, so it's best to keep some fresh lemons on hand. *Always* use freshly squeezed lemon juice from fresh lemons. *Never* use store-bought lemon juice, even if the juice says "freshly squeezed." You never know how fresh is fresh, and in what condition the lemons were prior to being processed.

A good practice is to purchase several fresh lemons when they are in season (and less expensive). Then you can squeeze them and freeze the juice in very small containers, half a cup or less, or in ice-cube trays. The frozen cubes can be removed and stored in a plastic freezer bag. That way, you will have freshly frozen squeezed lemon juice on hand for whatever purpose you need.

Matzah and Matzah Meal

Matzah is unleavened bread, traditionally eaten on the Jewish holiday of Passover (in the spring), but generally available all year around in most major metropolitan areas. Matzah comes in different varieties, including plain (white), egg and whole wheat. Matzah meal is matzah which has been ground up to produce very fine crumbs. Matzah meal is used in place of flour.

White matzah meal is available commercially.

Whole wheat matzah meal is not available commercially, but may be made very easily. Take a few boards of whole wheat matzah at a time. Break them into a blender or food processor and blend on high speed until the crumbs are sufficiently fine to use. This is a very noisy process, but takes little time.

Mochi Rice Thickener

This thickener is a very fine white rice flour that is used in place of cornstarch. If cornstarch is tolerated, you may substitute that for the rice flour through Stage I.

Nonfat, Non-instant Milk Powder

Nonfat, non-instant milk powder is a very thick type of milk powder that we use in some recipes. It is different from the type of milk powder generally available commercially, ("instant" milk powder) because non-instant milk powder is only heated once. Instant milk powder is heated twice. Non-instant milk powder retains much more flavor and sweetness than instant milk powder. This type of milk powder generally is available in health food stores and cooperatives.

Oil

We prefer safflower oil for cooking, although other oils may be acceptable on occasion, such as olive oil or canola oil.

When purchasing oil, you should pay careful attention to the method of extracting the oil from the plant. All vegetable oils are derived naturally through a process called "expeller pressing" or through a synthetic process using a petrochemical solvent. Expeller pressing involves putting seeds through a washing or steaming process, then pressing them, at low temperatures, to squeeze out the oils. The oil is then filtered to remove seed meal and bottled. These oils are labelled "expeller pressed" or "mechanically pressed" or "unrefined". Under current labelling laws, the manufacturer need not state the method of extraction.

We recommend only expeller pressed oil. First, synthetic extraction processes often use high heat and/or chemicals, which may cause cancer causing compounds to be formed. Second, adding chemicals is not necessarily beneficial to health.

We recommend using safflower oil because the safflower plant is less likely to be mold contaminated than corn or olive oil. Safflower oil also contains all of the essential fatty acids.

Safflower oil comes in several grades. You will find it in the store in colors ranging from a very dark gold to a very light gold. The darker the oil, the more robust the flavor. We prefer the lighter grades, which do not overpower the other ingredients in a dish.

Other people studying and writing about yeast free diets may differ from the recommendation to use safflower oil as the main oil. They do not believe safflower oil is bad. However, they prefer olive oil and canola oil.

Canola oil and olive oil even in this program may be used. However, experiment with the recipes, particularly cakes and cookies, for taste. All three oils taste completely different, and you may need to make some adjustments. Soy oil may also be used if you are certain that whomever is eating your food is not sensitive to soy.

Some oils are completely unacceptable. They are cottonseed oil and corn oil. Cottonseed oil is mold contaminated, and contains other poisons that have been shown to cause heart disease in animals. Corn oil should not be used because corn is often mold contaminated.

Other researchers have written about using other types of fats and oils, and their nutritional benefits. Some of the information they put forth may contradict some of the information in this book, but these are good references.

For a general reference, see Dr. William Crook's book, *The Yeast Connection Handbook.* Dr. Crook summarizes the results of such noted researchers as Dr. Sidney Baker, Dr. Leo Galland and Dr. Laura Stevens. Dr. Baker's book, *Detoxification and Healing*, and Dr. Udo Erasmus' book, *Fats that Heal and Fats that Kill* also discuss fats and oils. Finally, Dr. James Balch and Phyllis A. Balch have written a comprehensive guide to nutritional healing, *Prescription for Nutritional Healing.* For complete references to these books, see ***Appendix: Additional Resources.***

Oven Temperature

All oven temperatures are in degrees Fahrenheit ("F").

Pasta

If you tolerate gluten, you can use wheat pasta. We recommend whole wheat pasta, for the greater nutritional value.

Begin incorporating whole wheat pasta into your diet gradually, by starting with 1/4 whole wheat to 3/4 white pasta, then increase to 1/2 and 1/2, then to 3/4 whole wheat to 1/4 white, until you are used to the richer flavor and texture of the whole wheat pasta. Eventually you can use 100% whole wheat.

If you do not tolerate gluten, or if you just don't like the taste of whole wheat pasta, we recommend the Pastariso brand of rice-based pasta. This rice pasta is lighter than whole wheat pasta, but is made from equally nutritious brown rice.

The Pastariso brand is approved for use by people with Celiac disease and/or an intolerance to gluten products. Pastariso makes rice pasta in many different shapes and sizes. It generally is available in health food stores and food cooperatives, and can be ordered in less common styles, such as fettucine, spinach spaghetti, angel hair and vermicelli. For more information, write:

> Rice Innovations, Inc.
> 1773 Bayly Street
> Pickering, Ontario
> Canada, L1W 2Y7

Potatoes

Recipes in this book using potatoes generally specify which type of potato to use, mainly red, white rose and russet. The type of potato determines the texture and flavor of the dish. You can experiment with different types, of course, and you will add even more variety to your diet.

Red Potatoes are firmer than russet potatoes and have a sweet and crisp flavor when cooked. They tend to hold their shape better than russets.

White Rose Potatoes taste similar to red potatoes and have a similar texture, but are sweeter.

Russet Potatoes have a grainier texture, and are delicious baked or used in many of the dishes in this cookbook.

Purchase only the best quality potatoes. We strongly suggest buying potatoes individually rather than in prepackaged sacks, unless you get such a great deal from a farmer during growing season that you can afford to compost or throw out any bad potatoes.

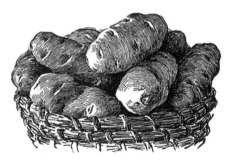

When you purchase bagged potatoes in the store, particularly at discount stores, you do not know what you are getting. Potatoes often have fungus or mold growths in them, which we see as a green layer directly under or on the skin, or brown or black spots under the skin or inside the potato.

Do not purchase or use potatoes that have become soft or

green, or which have actively growing sprouts. To ensure you are not eating bad spots, we recommend peeling the potatoes, cutting out any bad spots, then slicing the potatoes lengthwise and crosswise, and removing bad spots from the interior. Interior bad spots seem to be common in large russet potatoes.

Pumpkin

Recipes in this book turn out best by using fresh pumpkin. If necessary, use canned pumpkin, but this is not recommended. Pie pumpkins generally are available in the fall. They are small, sweet pumpkins. If pie pumpkins are not available, use the smaller standard pumpkins.

One small pumpkin (about 10 inches in diameter) generally makes enough pureed pumpkin for about two and a half cups of puree. Since pumpkins only seem to be available October and November, you can plan ahead and process several pumpkins, freezing or canning the extra for use later in the year.

Pumpkin can be prepared in the microwave oven, regular oven or on the stove. Microwaving takes less time and is easier, but you lose the seeds, which are delicious roasted and salted.

Microwave directions:

Place the whole pumpkin on a microwave safe plate and cook on high for 12 minutes. The pumpkin shell should pierce easily and the interior should be soft. If not, cook for another 2 minutes and test again.

Repeat in one minute intervals until pumpkin is tender. Then, let the pumpkin cool until you can handle it, cut in half, scoop out the seeds, then scoop out the edible pulp from the shell. Discard or compost the seeds and shell and proceed to pureeing directions.

Stove top or oven directions:

Cut the pumpkin in halves or quarters. Scoop out the seeds and the stringy material holding the seeds together. Set aside. Place the pieces of pumpkin shell side up in a large pot for steaming or on a greased cookie sheet for baking.

If steaming, add about half an inch of water to the pot and cover the pot. Bring the water to boil, then reduce to simmer for 30-60 minutes, until the pumpkin is fork tender. Let cool. Separate the soft interior from the hard, thin shell.

Preparing for use in recipes:
Puree the pumpkin in a food processor or a blender until very smooth. Pureed pumpkin can be frozen.

Pumpkin seeds:

Roasted pumpkin seeds are an added treat when you use fresh pumpkin. See the recipe in *Mainly Vegetables*.

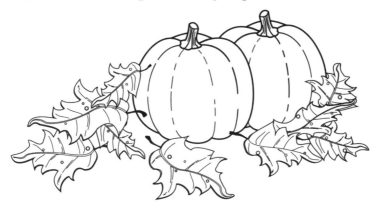

Rice

All recipes use raw, long-grained brown rice unless otherwise noted. We use brown rice instead of white rice because brown rice has much more nutritional value than white rice. The "brown" part of the brown rice is a thin outer covering that all rice naturally has. This covering contains some of the fiber, and all of the vitamins and minerals in the rice. To make white rice, processors remove this outer covering, along with the vitamins and minerals, as well as some fiber. Brown rice has a rich, nutty flavor. If you have never used brown rice, you are in for a treat!

To avoid family objections, begin by substituting brown rice for white rice slowly. Start with 1/4 cup of brown rice for every 3/4 cup of white rice (for 1 cup total), then increase to half and half, then to 3/4 brown rice for 1/4 white rice. After a few weeks, you will become accustomed to the different flavor and texture of brown rice.

Rice Mix

We use Ener-G brand rice mix for a few items. This is commonly available through health food stores and/or food cooperatives. If it is not available, write to :

Ener-G Foods
P.O. Box 84487
Seattle, WA 98124-5787

Salt

All of the recipes using salt call for sea salt rather than regular table salt. Sea salt tastes different because it is totally natural. Sea salt contains all of the minerals that you need, including iodine. Table salt contains additives such as dextrose, which is a sugar, and no minerals except in some cases added iodine. If you cannot get sea salt, you may substitute regular table salt, but be aware that the flavor of the recipe will be different. Add the salt a little at a time and taste before adding more.

Our recipes tend to be well salted. If you do not care for salt, or are on a severely restricted low sodium diet, use your common sense and start with less salt, adding salt to taste as you go.

Tomatoes

We use a lot of tomatoes, mainly because they are so delicious and they are one of the few foods our son tolerates well. I do not specify in the recipes to peel the tomatoes. This is because we do not mind small pieces of tomato skin in sauces and soups, and because peeling tomatoes takes much more time than I generally have to cook. However, if you like smoother foods, and/or you have more time available, peel your tomatoes before using them in any cooked recipe (soup or sauce, etcetera).

To peel tomatoes, do either of the following:

Using an open flame: hold the tomato (by a fork) over a hot flame. When the skin blisters, slip it off.

Using boiling water: Bring water to a boil in a large pot. Place two or three tomatoes in the boiling water. When the skin splits, remove the tomatoes at once and slip off the skins.

Water

The amounts of water given in these recipes are for standard cooking pots that allow some water to steam off. Only you know whether your cooking pots and pans require more or less water than standard recipes. If your pots are particularly tight, use less water when making things like steamed rice. If they leak a lot, you may need to add more water. The amount of water for soups and other watery dishes should be about the same as indicated in the recipes.

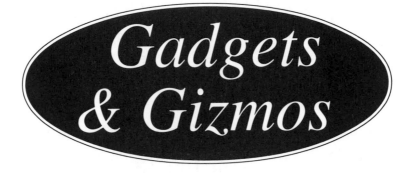

Gadgets & Gizmos

Healthy cooking takes time. So we rely heavily on tools to make the task faster and easier. This chapter suggests which types of cooking tools you may wish to stock to make your job easier!

Feasting without fermented food requires much more kitchen time and preparation than "ordinary" cooking. Virtually everything must be prepared fresh and from scratch, using no artificial ingredients. The only packaged ingredients used in this cookbook are pasta and some rice products. So, we are constantly looking for gadgets and gizmos to lessen our kitchen time. I (Lori) happen to love gadgets and buttons, so the more gadgets we have, the more fun cooking is.

Most recipes require tools that well equipped kitchens have, such as blenders. The only recipes requiring special tools are the ice cream and sorbet desserts, which use an ice cream maker.

In addition to your regular kitchen stock, these the gadgets will be helpful in your cooking:

Small appliances

Blender or food processor

A blender is a relatively inexpensive way to ensure that you are able to make most of the recipes in this book. A food processor will shorten your preparation time, but is more 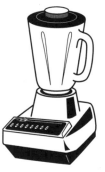 expensive. Either a blender or food processor is essential for making many of the soups and salad 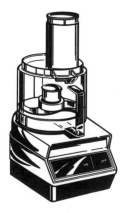 dressings, and all of the ice creams and sorbets. We use these tools to create creamy textures and to make sure that all ingredients are well mixed.

Deep Fryer

If you love french fries, invest in a small, inexpensive deep fryer (about 4 cup capacity). The french fries taste much better because they cook at the right heat, don't burn, and, most important to kids, look like restaurant french fries.

Electric skillet

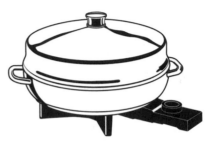

An electric skillet, or frying pan, creates another burner. This can be very helpful in a busy kitchen. The electric skillet also cooks food evenly at predictable temperatures. We use electric skillets primarily for all of our potato latke (pancake) recipes, and for our regular pancake recipes. You can also use an electric skillet instead of a wok.

Electric Mixer or Hand Mixer

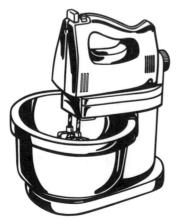

An electric mixer or hand mixer is useful for making cakes and blending other batters.

Ice Cream Maker

Desserts on a yeast/gluten/casein free diet are difficult to imagine without frozen sorbets and ice milks (for those who tolerate milk). We rely heavily on these desserts, summer and winter. Sorbet is a wonderful sweet and easy dessert that satisfies both children and adults. However, you cannot effectively duplicate the consistency of ice cream or store-bought sorbet without an ice cream maker. These small appliances are well worth the investment. We highly suggest that if you purchase an ice cream maker, you first get an electric one. Turning the hand crank is fun the first or second time, but you will think long and hard before making sorbet as a regular dessert!

We also advise purchasing an ice cream maker that uses a frozen cylinder rather than ice and salt. They are much less messy and are easier to use than the models requiring you to put in lots of ice and salt models. Their disadvantage is one is only able to make one batch of ice cream or sorbet every 12 hours.

Rice Steamer

Rice is an essential part of a yeast free, casein free and gluten free diet. Brown rice goes well with almost anything. Rice steamers help by cooking rice automatically, without the worry about burning it. There are many rice steamers on the market. Make sure you get one that is guaranteed to cook brown rice without presoaking. Many do not, or may say to soak the brown rice first. Do not soak the rice—this starts the fermentation process.

Slow Cooker

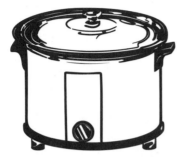

A 6-quart slow cooker is essential for a yeast free family. This is a small appliance that cooks food slowly and evenly, often over-night. We often have two in use at the same time. We recommend cooking beans in a slow cooker; many of our soup recipes are designed for a slow cooker. We find a slow cooker preferable to a "crock pot", because slow cookers are easier to clean (they are not as heavy). However, for cooking purposes, a 6 quart crock pot is fine.

Cooking Utensils

Baking Sheets

Two nonstick baking sheets are helpful for making cookies, as well as for freezing berries and roasting pumpkin seeds. We find the most useful type are the ones with a layer of air sand-wiched between two sheets of metal.

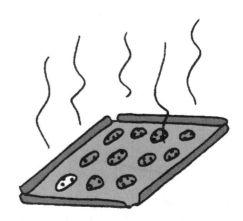

Cookware

A good set of pots and pans helps every good cook become a great cook. A poor set of pots and pans can make a good cook work much harder, because they allow foods to burn more easily. Bad pots and pans can also lend unwanted flavors to food. At a minimum, you will need a 3-quart and a 6-quart kettle (large stove top pot with a cover) to make many of the recipes in this book.

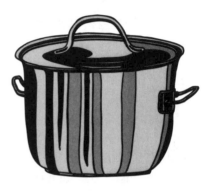

If you are replacing pots and pans, look for ones that conduct and hold heat well, and do not allow much water to escape during cooking. There are many excellent brands available. We prefer heavy, stainless steel pots and pans that have layers of iron and aluminum inside. Do not purchase aluminum cookware.

Wok

A wok is a Chinese cooking vessel that helps sear and cook foods very quickly at very high heat. Many of the recipes in this book are stir-fry recipes which you can cook much more easily in a wok.

Woks are available in virtually all department and cooking stores. If you live near a Chinese grocery store, get one there.

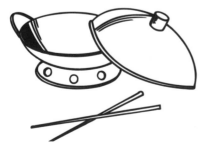

Woks come in both stove-top and electric models. We prefer the stove-top model, which cooks at a hotter temperature. Be sure you get a flat bottom for a electric stove and a rounded bottom with a stand for a gas stove.

Hand Tools

Grater

An old fashioned 4 sided grater is essential for making some of the potato recipes, such as **Hash Browns** and all of the potato latke (pancake) recipes. For reasons we do not quite understand, grated potatoes do not come out the same using a food processor.

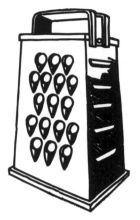

Knives

Good knives are essential for a well equipped kitchen. Chinese cleavers work best for chopping, especially vegetables. Make sure you have a simple knife sharpener or sharpening stone on hand, and that you use it frequently!

Pastry Blender

This is a small hand too that significantly shortens the time involved in making pie crust and other things that require chopping. We use ours a lot!

Whisk

A whisk is another small hand tool useful for blending foods together quickly.

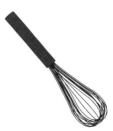

Bon Appetit!

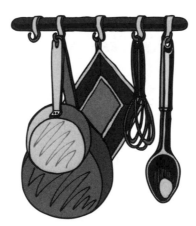

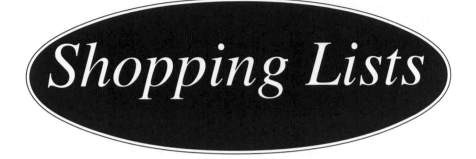

Shopping Lists

Using a master shopping list can simplify life on a yeast free diet. You can photocopy the lists in this chapter to use as checkoffs, or just keep a copy with you, so you always have the basic foods on hand for just about any recipe in this book. List 1 gives basic supplies for most recipes in this book. List 2 adds some packaged products, fruit, fish, poultry and beef. List 3 adds dairy and wheat.

If you are following the Stages, the lists are presented in reverse order of the diet. List 1, the Basic List, corresponds to all recipes suitable through Stage IV. List 2 builds on List 1, and corresponds to Stage III. If you are following Stage IV, then, all you need to use is List 1. If you are on Stage III, you will need Lists 1 and 2. List 3 adds more foods, including wheat and milk, and corresponds to Stages I and II. If you are on Stage I or II, you will need all three lists.

List 1

To Shop, for Stage IV, use just this list. For Stage III, use this list plus List 2; for Stages I and II, use this list, plus Lists 2 and 3

☐ Dried Beans (Black, Navy, Kidney, Lentils)

☐ Long Grained Brown Rice

☐ Unprocessed Clover Honey

☐ Expeller Pressed Safflower Oil

☐ Sea Salt

☐ Rice Cakes (Brown Rice and Salt, or unsalted)

☐ Rice Pasta (Pastariso Brand)

☐ Hot Rice cereal

☐ Dried Herbs

☐ Ener-G brand Rice Mix

☐ Brown Rice Flour

☐ Meat: veal and/or lamb; occasional turkey or chicken (hormone/antibiotic free)

☐ Eggs (if possible, get "farm fresh" eggs without hormones or antibiotics)

☐ Butter

Produce:

☐ Fresh berries in season (blueberries, raspberries, cranberries, blackberries, but not strawberries)

☐ Fresh herbs, when available, including basil, dill, oregano, parsley, and others

☐ Fresh Vegetables, including: bok choy, broccoli, cabbage, carrots, celery, cubanel pepper (mild pepper), green beans, green pepper, sweet red pepper, kohlrabi, lettuce, zucchini and other summer squash; pumpkins and winter squash

☐ Leeks, scallions or spring onions

☐ Lemons

☐ Potatoes: russet, red, white rose, yukon gold, whatever looks good

☐ Sweet Potatoes

☐ Tomatoes

List 2

To Shop, for Stages I-III, use this list plus List 1; for Stages I and II, use this list, plus Lists 1 and 3

☐ Canned Tuna Fish (labelled "very low sodium"--only ingredients Tuna Fish and Water)

☐ Meats: Poultry, Beef

☐ Packaged cereals without wheat/gluten, such as Puffed Rice, Puffed Millet and Puffed Corn

☐ Ice cream substitutes, such as "Rice Dream" (rice based) brand and/or "Tofutti" (soy based), but without chocolate and/or nuts

☐ Chips, if cooked in appropriate oil (not cottonseed or peanut; soy oil, canola, safflower are acceptable).

☐ Fresh Fish

☐ Fresh Fruit: any fresh fruit except apples and grapes, including pears, oranges, tangerines, grapefruit, melons, mangoes, papaya, etc., unless you cannot tolerate that fruit for some other reason.

Check all labels on all packaged products to ensure nothing (1) contains the word "malt", including barley malt, malted barley flour, maltodextrin, etc.; (2) contains cottonseed oil or cottonseed meal; (3) contains vinegar.

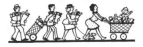

List 3

To Shop, for Stages I and II, use this list plus Lists 1 and 2

☐ Commercial cereals, made without malt: at the time of publication, "General Mills" did not use malt in most of its cereals, including Cheerios, Kix, and Total. HOWEVER, *check each label to be sure the manufacturer has not changed the ingredients since the last time you purchased the product.*

☐ Commercial chips, crackers, etc., made without malt, cottonseed or peanut products

☐ Oatmeal

☐ Milk

☐ For Stage I-A: apples and grapes

☐ Whole Wheat tortillas or chapatis

☐ Whole Wheat pasta

☐ Whole Wheat flour (check to be sure no malt has been added to the flour)

☐ Unbleached white flour, if preferred for some recipes (check to be sure no malt has been added to the flour. Most commercial white flours use malt)

☐ Whole Wheat Pastry Flour

☐ Whole wheat bread without malt

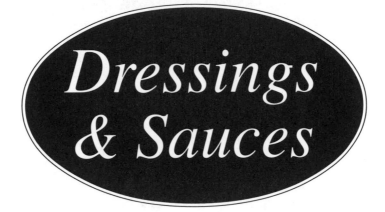

Dressings & Sauces

Salsas, pasta sauces, salad dressings and other dips make meals more festive. This chapter provides many recipes for delicious:

    ~ Salad Dressings

    ~ Pasta Sauces

    ~ Fruit Sauces

    ~ Salsas & Dips

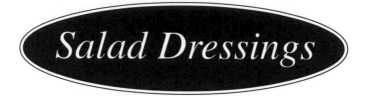

Lemon Herb Salad Dressing

Cholesterol Free
Wheat/Gluten Free
Milk/Casein Free
Egg Free
Suitable through Stage IV

Delightfully light and flavorful, this dressing is a great substitute
for any vinaigrette dressing and can be used on all salads.

1/2 c. freshly squeezed lemon juice

2/3 c. expeller pressed safflower oil

1/2 tsp. dried basil

1/2 tsp. dried oregano

1/2 tsp. dried thyme flakes

1/2 tsp. dried dill

1/2 tsp. dried marjoram

1 tsp. sea salt

1/2 c. water

Mix all ingredients in a small container with a lid. Shake well.
Refrigerate at least 2 hours before use. This dressing keeps well
in the refrigerator for only about 2 days, but may be frozen. For
convenience, freeze in an ice cube tray and defrost one or two
cubes at a time. Makes about 1-1/2 c. dressing.

Creamy Cucumber Dressing

> *Cholesterol Free*
> *Wheat/Gluten Free*
> *Milk/Casein Free*
> *Egg Free*
> *Suitable through Stage IV*

This salad dressing is the most popular dressing we serve. It goes well with salads of all types, as well as with fish or vegetables.

    1 large cucumber

    2 T. fresh dill weed, or 5 tsp. dried dill weed

    1/2-1 tsp. sea salt, or salt to taste

    1 T. freshly squeezed lemon juice

    1/3 c. expeller pressed safflower oil

Peel and chop the cucumber into chunks. Place all ingredients in blender. Blend thoroughly. Serve fresh or chilled. This dressing is great on salads, vegetables, fish or just about anything else. It refrigerates well for about a day. Freeze any extra and defrost as needed.

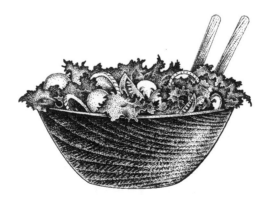

Tomato Garlic Dressing

> *Cholesterol Free*
> *Wheat/Gluten Free*
> *Milk/Casein Free*
> *Egg Free*
> *Suitable through Stage IV*

This dressing has a creamy consistency and is very tasty. Use it when you want to perk up a meal!

1 large or 2 small tomatoes

1 large or 2 small cloves garlic

1-1/2 tsp. dried oregano

1/2 tsp. sea salt

1/3 c. expeller pressed safflower oil

Chop the tomato into chunks. Peel the garlic and microwave for 1 minute on "high." Place the oil in a blender and add the oregano and salt. *Blend* on high for a short time, until blended. Add the garlic. Then gradually add the chunks of tomato. Continue blending until the mixture is completely smooth. Serve immediately or chilled. If chilled, mix well before serving. If you have any extra, keep in the refrigerator for up to a day, or freeze.

Creamy Tomato Herb Salad Dressing

> *Cholesterol Free*
> *Wheat/Gluten Free*
> *Milk/Casein Free*
> *Egg Free*
> *Suitable through Stage IV*

This is easy, fast and tasty, and great for dipping vegetables, too.

1/3 c. expeller pressed safflower oil

1 large or two medium tomatoes

1-1/2 tsp. dried tarragon *or* basil *or* oregano

1 to 1-1/2 tsp. sea salt

Chop the tomato(es). ***Choose your herbs*** according to your taste: tarragon is sweet; oregano is sharp; basil is somewhere between the two. ***Combine*** all ingredients in a blender or food processor. For the salt, begin with 1/2 tsp., then taste after blending. Blend on high until the dressing is very smooth and creamy. It should not be grainy. Add extra salt if desired. Delicious! If you have leftovers, you can keep this in the refrigerator for a day, or freeze it.

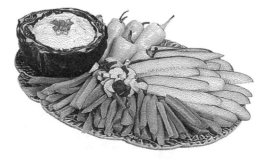

Sarah's Zucchini Salad Dressing

Cholesterol Free
Wheat/Gluten Free
Milk/Casein Free
Egg Free
Suitable through Stage IV

1 large tomato, or 2 small tomatoes

1 large or 2 small zucchini

1 clove garlic

1 tsp. sea salt

1/2 tsp. dried oregano

1/4 tsp. dried marjoram

1/4 tsp. dried thyme

1 tsp. unprocessed clover honey

6 T. water

Chop the tomatoes, zucchini and garlic. Place all ingredients in blender. Blend on highest speed until really liquid. Chill and serve. Freeze extra in ice cube trays and use as needed.

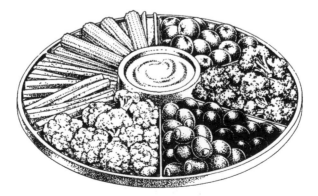

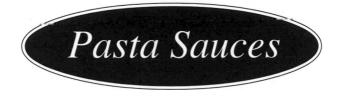

Pasta Sauces

Fresh Basil and Tomato Sauce

> *Cholesterol Free (using oil)*
> *Wheat/Gluten Free*
> *Milk/Casein Free*
> *Egg Free*
> *Suitable through Stage IV*

Few herbs are tastier than fresh sweet basil at the end of August. We make this sauce in large quantities (two or three batches at a time) and freeze it for later use. This sauce is very rich; a little goes a long way. Don't skimp on the butter! One batch is enough for pasta sauce for 5-6 hungry people.

    3 large tomatoes

    1 c. packed fresh basil leaves

    3 T. butter *or* expeller pressed safflower oil

    1 tsp. sea salt, or salt to taste

Heat a skillet on medium heat. While the skillet is heating, *chop* the tomatoes into chunks. Chop the basil leaves into smaller pieces. When the skillet is hot, *melt* the butter or heat the oil. Throw in the basil leaves and cook about a minute, until they are soft. Add the tomatoes and salt. Cook until the tomatoes form a sauce, at least 15 minutes. If you like chunky sauce, mash down the tomatoes and serve as is. If you prefer a smoother, creamier sauce, puree in a blender until smooth, then serve over "Pastariso" brand rice pasta. This sauce freezes well.

Fiesta Fettucine Sauce

> *Cholesterol Free (using oil)*
> *Wheat/Gluten Free*
> *Milk/Casein Free*
> *Egg Free*
> *Suitable through Stage IV*

This pasta dish is delicious and fun to serve. It tastes best over brown rice fettucine (Pastariso brand), or whole wheat fettucine (if you tolerate gluten).

   2 boxes (approx. 20 oz.) "Pastariso" brand brown rice fettucine *or* whole wheat fettucine

   2 T. butter *or* 2 T. expeller pressed safflower oil

   4 c. chopped mixed bell peppers (red, yellow, green)

   1 lb. asparagus

   2 T. fresh dill weed

   1/2 tsp. sea salt + more to taste

Cook the pasta according to package directions. When pasta is done, drain and place in a large serving bowl. *While the pasta is cooking, cook the sauce, as follows*:   Heat the butter or oil in a large skillet. When the butter has melted or the oil is hot, saute the bell pepper. *Chop* the asparagus into one inch lengths, discarding the tough ends. Add the asparagus and dill weed to the bell peppers, saute until vegetables are soft and cooked through. Add salt, starting with 1/2 tsp., then adding more to taste. *Mix* the sauce through the pasta. Serve immediately.

Fresh Pizza Tomato Sauce

Wheat/Gluten Free
Milk/Casein Free
Egg Free
Suitable through Stage IV

Fresh basil and oregano at the end of the summer combine to make an outstanding pizza sauce that can be served on pizza, pasta or just about anything else. This is a very rich sauce; a little goes a long way.

   1/2 c. packed fresh basil leaves

   1/2 c. packed fresh oregano leaves

   5 large tomatoes

   3 T. butter

   1 tsp. sea salt, or salt to taste

Heat a skillet on medium heat. While the skillet is heating, ***chop*** the tomatoes into chunks. Chop the herbs into smaller pieces. When the skillet is hot, melt the butter. Throw in the herbs and cook about a minute, until they are soft. ***Add*** the tomatoes and salt. ***Cook*** until the tomatoes form a sauce, at least 15 minutes. If you like chunky sauce, mash down the tomatoes and serve as is. If you prefer a smoother, creamier, thicker sauce, puree in a blender until smooth, then serve over "Pastariso" brand rice pasta. This sauce freezes well.

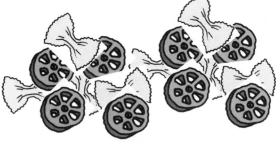

Creamy Herb Sauce

Egg Free
Suitable through Stage II

This is a different type of pasta sauce, not dependent on tomatoes for flavor. The sauce is delicious over pasta, rice or vegetables If you are gluten intolerant, see the recipe for *Fresh Herb Sauce.*

3 T. butter

1/4 c. chopped fresh oregano, *or* 1 T. dried oregano

1/4 c. chopped fresh basil, *or* 1 T. dried basil

2 large cloves garlic, chopped

2 T. whole wheat pastry flour

1-1/2 c. liquid: use nonfat milk, liquid from steamed vegetables,and/or water in whatever proportions you have available or desire

1/2 tsp. sea salt, or salt to taste

Melt the butter in a sauce pan. Briefly *saute* the garlic and dried herbs for 1-2 minutes. If using fresh herbs, you will add them later. On medium heat, quickly *stir or whisk* the flour into the butter. *Add* the liquid in small amounts, being careful to stir or whisk it in completely before adding more. When all the liquid has been added, continue to stir frequently until the sauce thickens. *Add* the fresh herbs. Salt to taste. Let the sauce sit a few minutes to absorb the flavors prior to serving.

Fresh Herb Sauce

Wheat/Gluten Free
Egg Free
Milk/Casein Free
Suitable through Stage IV

This is a deliciously delicate and tasty sauce that can be served over pasta or rice. Guests give it rave reviews. This can be prepared close to serving time, if you are in a hurry, or several hours in advance, if you prefer to let the flavors simmer together.

6 T. butter

5 large cloves garlic

1/4 c. fresh, chopped oregano, *or* 1 T. dried oregano

1/4 c. fresh, chopped basil, *or* 1 T. dried basil

optional: fresh dill, fresh rosemary

2 sweet red bell peppers

2 ripe tomatoes

1 green and/or yellow bell pepper *(optional)*

sea salt to taste

1-1/2 lbs. whole wheat *or* brown rice pasta, cooked according to package directions

Melt the butter in a large skillet. *Chop* the garlic. *Add* the garlic and herbs to the melted butter. This tastes best with fresh herbs, but dried herbs may be used. While the herbs are cooking, *chop* the peppers and tomatoes. *Add* the peppers and tomatoes to the herbs and saute for a few minutes, until the peppers are soft.   Add salt to taste. You now are ready to serve. A little bit of this sauce goes a long way. Mix a little with each plate of pasta, or mix the entire amount into one to 1-1/2 lbs. of cooked whole wheat spaghetti or fettucine or the equivalent amount of rice pasta.

Quick 'N Easy Tomato Sauce

> *Cholesterol Free*
> *Wheat/Gluten Free*
> *Milk/Casein Free*
> *Egg Free*
> *Suitable through Stage IV*

This sauce is so quick and easy that it is close to being "fast food." The recipe takes about 5 minutes to make, start to finish, if your pan is hot enough. This recipe makes enough for about 6 servings—just enough for lunch. Kids love it mixed with rice pasta. We find that serving the sauce on top of the pasta doesn't work—the kids just eat the sauce!   Do not cut back on the oil and butter. The rich flavor makes a little sauce go a long way. If you don't like pasta, this sauce is terrific mixed into rice.

    2 medium tomatoes

    1 T. butter

    1 T. expeller pressed safflower oil

    1 tsp. dried basil

    1 tsp. dried oregano

    1 tsp. sea salt

Heat a skillet on the stove on medium heat. While the skillet is heating, *chop* the tomatoes. Set the tomatoes aside. When the skillet is hot, *melt* the butter. *Add* the oil. Heat until hot. *Add* the tomatoes. These will fall apart and form a sauce with the butter and oil. *Add* the basil, oregano and salt. Cook through. If desired, *mash* the tomatoes with a potato masher or, for thicker, smoother sauce, *puree* in a blender. Serve over "Pastariso" brand rice pasta. *Variation*: Add a sweet red bell pepper while you are cooking the tomatoes. This gives the sauce a fresh and crunchy consistency and sweetens the flavor. Makes 6 servings for hungry people.

Tomato, Dill and Marjoram Sauce

Wheat/Gluten Free
Egg Free
Milk/Casein Free (with butter)
Suitable through Stage IV

Like all great recipes, this one started out as a mistake, using only ingredients we had on hand at the time at a lake cottage where we had forgotten to bring seasonings. This is one of the most popular sauces we make and disappears immediately. It's great over pasta, rice pasta, plain rice or just about anything else.

2 T. butter

2 very large beefsteak tomatoes *or* 4 medium tomatoes

1 tsp. dried dill

1 tsp. dried marjoram

1 T. unprocessed clover honey

1 tsp. sea salt

Melt the butter in a large skillet. Chop the tomatoes while the butter is melting. Add the chopped tomatoes, herbs and salt. *Bring to a boil*, cover, and simmer for at least 30 minutes. The longer you cook it, the better it tastes. *Mix;* while you are mixing, mash the tomatoes. Add the honey. If the sauce is too thick, add some water. If the sauce is to thin, remove the cover and boil a few minutes to evaporate the excess liquid. If thicker, smoother sauce is desired, *puree* the sauce in a blender prior to serving. Serve hot.

Sweet Pepper Pasta Sauce With Beans

Cholesterol Free
Wheat/Gluten Free
Milk/Casein Free
Egg Free
Suitable through Stage IV

This is a tasty, chunky sweet red pepper sauce. It is best served over pasta (or rice pasta), but is also great over potatoes or rice. The sauce freezes well. This sauce takes at least three hours to simmer to full flavor, and tastes best if you start it early in the day.

2 T. expeller pressed safflower oil for sauteing

5-6 cloves garlic, minced

4 medium zucchini, sliced

2 sweet red bell peppers, chopped

1 large eggplant, peeled and cubed

1 quart home canned tomatoes, or 6 large tomatoes, peeled and diced

1 T. dried basil

1 T. dried oregano

1 T. sea salt (or sea salt to taste)

2-1/2 c. dry beans, cooked according to directions in *Mainly Beans,* including draining and rinsing

 In a large (6 quart) kettle, *heat* safflower oil . *Add* garlic, being careful not to burn. Add zucchini; saute a few minutes. Add red bell peppers; saute. Then add the eggplant, sauteing. Add the herbs and salt. *Cover and let cook* down for 1/2 hour or so on low heat. When the eggplant is soft and cooked through, *add* the tomatoes. *Add* the beans. Bring the entire mixture up to a boil, then turn to low heat and simmer for 2 hours or more. Test for salt and add if necessary. Serve hot.

Fresh Basil Butter Sauce

Wheat/Gluten Free
Milk/Casein Free
Egg Free
Suitable through Stage IV

This "sauce" is just basil and butter—a little goes a long way.

    1/2 c. butter

    1/2 c. chopped fresh basil

Melt the butter in a saucepan. When it sizzles, add the chopped basil. Cook through until the basil is still bright, but soft and wilted. Serve in small quantities mixed through rice pasta, brown rice, or on a baked potato. Enjoy!

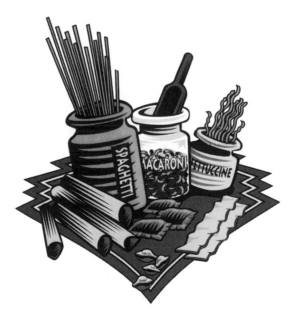

Pesto

Cholesterol Free
Wheat/Gluten Free
Milk/Casein Free
Egg Free
Suitable through Stage IV

This nontraditional pesto uses basil as its flavoring and zucchini as a filler. It is lighter than traditional pesto, which uses cheese and pine nuts. Serve in small (1-2 T.) servings over pasta, then mix through.

1-1/4 c. grated zucchini

1/2 c. expeller pressed safflower oil

1 tsp. sea salt

1 c. packed fresh basil leaves

In a blender, puree the zucchini and oil. Add the salt and mix. Add the basil leaves one fourth at a time. Chop. For a smoother consistency, puree. If not using immediately, freeze in ice cube trays and defrost as needed. Makes about 1-1/2 cups.

Fresh Oregano Dill Sauce

> *Cholesterol Free*
> *Wheat/Gluten Free*
> *Milk/Casein Free*
> *Egg Free*
> *Suitable through Stage IV*

2 leeks

2 cloves garlic

9 medium tomatoes

2 T. expeller pressed safflower oil

1/3 c. packed fresh oregano leaves

1/4 c. packed fresh dill weed

Thoroughly **wash and chop** the leeks, using as much green as possible. Mince the garlic. Chop the tomatoes and set aside. Heat a large frying pan. **Heat** the oil in the pan. When the oil is hot, **add** the leeks and garlic. **Saute** until the leeks are soft. Add the herbs. Saute until wilted. Add the tomatoes. **Saute** until the tomatoes are soft and mushy. Serve as is, or, for a thicker sauce, puree in a blender or food processor.

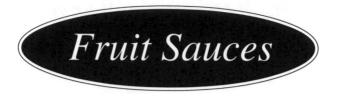

Cranberry Pear Sauce

> *Cholesterol Free*
> *Wheat/Gluten Free*
> *Milk/Casein Free*
> *Egg Free*
> *Suitable through Stage III*

This is a delicious variation of the Thanksgiving cranberry sauce with which I grew up. If pears are not tolerated, use the **Cranberry Lemon Sauce** .

1 pkg. fresh cranberries (about 2-3 cups)

1-1/2 c. unprocessed clover honey

2 medium to large fresh pears

Peel and chop the pears. ***Mix*** all ingredients in a three quart saucepan. Cover; bring to a slow boil; reduce to simmer. With the top ajar or off altogether, ***simmer*** for 45 minutes to an hour, stirring occasionally. Remove from heat. Cool to room temperature while uncovered, then store in refrigerator until ready to use.   Freezes well. Makes about 3-4 cups.

Cranberry Lemon Sauce

> *Cholesterol Free*
> *Wheat/Gluten Free*
> *Milk/Casein Free*
> *Egg Free*
> *Suitable through Stage IV*

This is a delicious fresh cranberry sauce, tolerated by even the most sensitive people.

    2 packages fresh cranberries (about 4-6 c.)

    2 c. unprocessed clover honey, plus more to taste

    2 fresh lemons

Pour the cranberries and honey in a 3 quart pot on low heat. Slice the lemons, including peel, very thin. Add to the cranberries and mix. Cover; bring to a slow boil; reduce to *simmer*. With the top ajar or off altogether, simmer for 45 minutes to an hour, stirring occasionally. Remove from heat. *Cool* to room temperature while uncovered, then store in refrigerator until ready to use.   Freezes well. Makes about 2-3 cups.

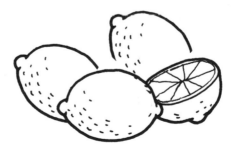

Cranberry Fruit Sauce

> *Cholesterol Free*
> *Wheat/Gluten Free*
> *Milk/Casein Free*
> *Egg Free*
> *Suitable through Stage III*

This is a delicious variation of the Thanksgiving cranberry sauce with which I grew up. The citrus fruit gives this sauce a sweet and sour flavor. If oranges and/or pears are not tolerated, use *Cranberry Lemon Sauce*.

    1 pkg. fresh cranberries   (about 3-4 c.)

     1-1/2 c. unprocessed clover honey

    2 medium to large fresh pears

    1 lemon in season

    1 orange in season

Peel and chop the pears. Slice the lemon and orange, leaving the peel on. *Mix* all ingredients in a three quart saucepan. *Cover* the pan and bring to a slow boil; reduce to simmer. With the top ajar or off altogether, *simmer* for 45 minutes to an hour, stirring occasionally. Remove from heat. *Cool* to room temperature while uncovered, then store in refrigerator until ready to use.   Freezes well. Makes about 3-4 cups.

Haroset for Passover

> *Cholesterol Free*
> *Wheat/Gluten Free (without Matzah)*
> *Milk/Casein Free*
> *Egg Free*
> *Suitable through Stage IV*

Haroset is a traditional food that symbolizes an important part of Jewish history and has an integral role in the Passover Seder. Haroset, traditionally made from chopped apples, walnuts and wine, resembles the mortar used to build the pyramids during the 400 years when Jews were enslaved in Egypt. To maintain the symbolism and important part of Jewish history and religion, I devised a haroset that even our son could eat. Not only is this symbolic, it is delicious! This is a great fruit sauce, even if you are not Jewish.

  4 firm pears

  1/2 c. unprocessed honey

  1/2 c. water

  5 whole cloves

  1/2 tsp. cinnamon (optional)

  optional: 2 boards whole wheat matzah (contains gluten)

Peel and chop the pears into small pieces. Set aside. Bring honey, water, cloves and cinnamon to a *boil* in a small saucepan. Turn off heat. Add the pears. If using matzah, break into small pieces and *add* while sauce is still hot. Place in a serving dish and *refrigerate* until you are ready to use it. Refrigerates well for two days. Makes 4-6 cups.

Pear Sauce

Cholesterol Free
Gluten Free
Casein Free
Egg Free
Suitable through Stage III

This is an excellent sauce on its own, but also serves as a filling for **Hamantaschen Dough**, or served with any of the **Latke** recipes in **Mainly Potatoes**.

  5 firm pears

  2 T. unprocessed clover honey

  1/4 tsp. cinnamon

  2 whole cloves

  1/4 c. water

Peel and chop the pears into half inch cubes. Place all ingredients into a pot. Bring to a boil. Cover and simmer until pears are very soft. Stir. Press the pears to mash them up to make a sauce. If the mixture is too watery, remove the cover and let excess liquid boil off. Let cool, then eat or use to fill **Hamantaschen Dough**.

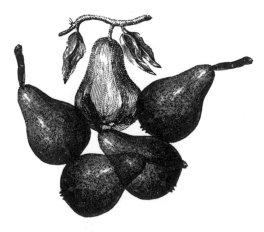

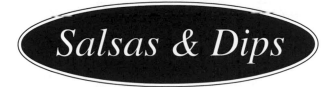

Hummus

Cholesterol Free
Wheat/Gluten Free
Milk/Casein Free
Egg Free
Suitable through Stage IV

Hummus is a good spread and dip and a tasty alternative to peanut butter.

3 cloves garlic

2 c. cooked garbanzo beans (chick peas)

1/2 c. expeller pressed safflower oil

1-1/2 tsp. sea salt

2 T. freshly squeezed lemon juice

Place the garlic, in their peels, in a small bowl. Microwave on high for 30 seconds. Set aside. When cool enough to handle, slip the garlic out of their skins. ***Place the oil*** in a blender or food processor. Add one cup of the beans. Puree until mixed, but slightly chunky. Add the second cup of beans, plus two cloves garlic. ***Puree*** until smooth. Add the salt, lemon juice, and third clove garlic. Puree until smooth or desired consistency. Serve immediately or refrigerate until ready to serve. Makes 2-3 cups of hummus.

Almost Barbecue Sauce

Cholesterol Free
Wheat/Gluten Free
Milk/Casein Free
Egg Free
Suitable through Stage IV

This sweet, sour, and slightly hot sauce closely resembles barbecue sauce. It tastes great with anything and everything on which you would use barbecue sauce.

> 2 c. cooked tomatoes (about 4 large tomatoes)
>
> 4 T. freshly squeezed lemon juice
>
> 3 T. unprocessed clover honey
>
> 1 tsp. sea salt
>
> 1/8 tsp. ground black pepper
>
> 1/2 tsp. dried basil
>
> 1/4 tsp. dried sage

Mix all ingredients in a one quart saucepan. Bring to a boil, then reduce to simmer. Simmer for 30 minutes, then let sit for an hour or more to allow the flavors to blend. Serve warm or cold. Makes about 1-1/2 to 2 cups of sauce.

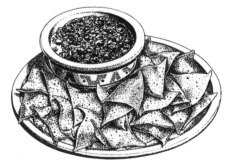

Sweet Super Bowl Salsa

> *Cholesterol Free*
> *Wheat/Gluten Free*
> *Milk/Casein Free*
> *Egg Free*
> *Suitable through Stage IV*

Hard to watch football without salsa? This is a delicious sweet pepper salsa. It does not contain hot peppers, but has enough zing to taste great at parties or as a snack. Our daughter Sarah created it for the 1997 Super Bowl, featuring the Green Bay Packers (hence the green and yellow peppers), and recommends it for kids who don't like spicy foods but like to eat salsa.

1/3 green bell pepper

1/3 yellow bell pepper

1/3 sweet red bell pepper

3 plum tomatoes

1 large clove garlic

1-1/2 tsp. dried oregano

salt to taste

1/2 c. water

2 T. freshly squeezed lemon juice

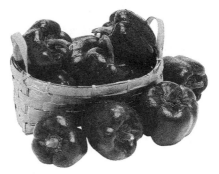

Chop the peppers and tomatoes. **Mince** the garlic. Place all ingredients in a one quart pot. **Heat** to boiling, then reduce to simmer. Let the mixture cook at least half an hour, until the peppers are soft. Remove from heat. If you just can't wait, enjoy the salsa right away. But the flavors will mingle and deepen if you chill the salsa an hour or two before serving. Makes about 1-1/2 cups.

Salsa Picante

Cholesterol Free
Wheat/Gluten Free
Milk/Casein Free
Egg Free
Suitable through Stage IV
(using mild chili peppers)
Suitable through Stage III
(using any chili peppers)

Craving spicy foods? This salsa is for you. This salsa can be mild or very spicy hot, depending on the type of peppers used.

1/3 c. chopped sweet red bell pepper

2 tsp. oregano

2 tomatoes

2 T. expeller pressed safflower oil

1 tsp. sea salt

for <u>mild</u> salsa: 1 T. chopped Cubanel chili pepper

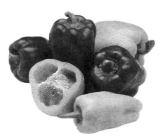

for <u>hot</u> salsa: up to 1 tsp. chopped fresh hot pepper (jalapeno or other)

Chop the tomatoes and set aside.
Heat the oil in a small saucepan.
When hot, *add* the other ingredients except the peppers. If using jalapeno or other very spicy peppers, add a little at a time and taste frequently to make sure you don't over spice the salsa. *Cook* on medium heat for 10 minutes or more. Let sit at least 30 minutes, to allow the flavor to settle. Enjoy!

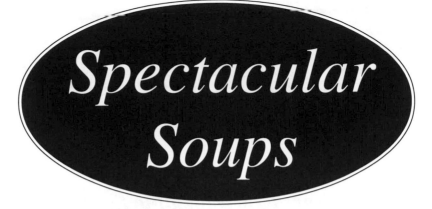

Spectacular Soups

We serve soups all year round. They are the mainstay of our menus. Most of the recipes in this chapter are designed for 6-quart pots or slow cookers. A few recipes are designed for 3-quart pots. The larger 6-quart recipes yield approximately 15 average sized servings (about 1-1/2 c.). This is usually enough for 8-10 people, including seconds. The 3-quart recipes make enough for 4-5 people. So have pots on hand and start cooking. . .

- ~ *Slow Cooking Soups*
- ~ *Cholents (rich, slow cooked stews)*
- ~ *Soups for Dumplings*
- ~ *Soothing Soups*
- ~ *Lentil Soups*
- ~ *Split Pea Soups*
- ~ *Creamy Soups*

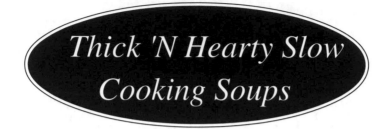

Tarragon Vegetable Soup

> *Cholesterol Free*
> *Wheat/Gluten Free (using rice)*
> *Milk/Casein Free*
> *Egg Free*
> *Suitable through Stage IV*

Sweet and fresh summer herbs give this soup a special taste. This is best made in a slow cooker, but can be made on the stove top. Start the night before and serve this soup for lunch or dinner the next day. The barley thickens the soup, but rice should be used for Wheat/Gluten Free soup.

3 lg. or 4 medium kohlrabi, peeled and diced

1/2 bunch celery (with tops left on), chopped

4 carrots, peeled and chopped

1/2 c. hulled barley *or* 1/2 c. brown rice

1/2 c. white beans (Navy or Great Northern)

1 tsp. dried rosemary, crushed between your fingers

3 tsp. dried basil

2 tsp. dried tarragon

5 whole black peppercorns (optional)

1 tsp. lemon thyme

1-2 T. sea salt, to taste

Optional: 1 qt. home-canned tomatoes, or 5 fresh tomatoes, peeled and chopped

10-14 c. water

Combine all ingredients except water in a 6-quart kettle or a 6-quart slow cooker. Fill with enough water to within half an inch of the top, usually 10-14 cups. Cover. If using the stove top method, bring to a boil, then reduce to simmer and cook for at least two hours, or until the beans are thoroughly cooked. If using the slow cooker, turn to "high" and cook several hours or overnight, then reduce to low to keep warm. Check water periodically, and add more if necessary. Serve piping hot!

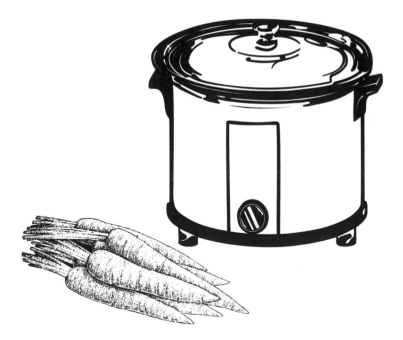

Summer Black-Eyed Pea Soup

Cholesterol Free
Milk/Casein Free
Egg Free
Suitable through Stage II

Fresh oregano and basil balance the spicy black-eyed peas to give this soup the heartiness of fall with the tangy taste of summer. This should be started several hours before serving, and can be made in a slow cooker.

1 c. dry black-eyed peas

1 c. hulled barley

4 carrots, peeled and chopped

2 zucchini, sliced

2 c. fresh green beans, sliced

3 medium kohlrabi, peeled and cubed

1 quart home-canned tomatoes, including juice *or* 5 large fresh tomatoes, chopped

large handful of fresh oregano leaves, chopped

1 T. dried basil or 1/4 c. packed fresh basil leaves, chopped

6 black peppercorns (optional)

1-2 T. sea salt, to taste

10-14 c. water

Place all ingredients except water in a 6-quart slow cooker or kettle with enough water to come within 1/2 inch of the top of the pot, usually about 10-14 cups. *Cover.* If using the stove top method, bring to a boil, then reduce to simmer and cook for at least two hours, or until the beans are thoroughly cooked. If using the slow cooker, turn to "high" and cook several hours or overnight, then reduce to low to keep warm. Check water periodically, and add more if necessary. Serve as soon as the beans are soft enough to eat.

Zesty Barley Bean Soup

Cholesterol Free
Milk/Casein Free
Egg Free
Suitable through Stage II

This soup takes out the winter chills, with a little zip for extra energy. Start early in the day, or the night before.

8 medium fresh tomatoes, or 1 one-quart jar home canned tomatoes, chopped

4 stalks celery, including leaves, chopped

3 medium or 2 large kohlrabi, peeled and diced

4 carrots, peeled and chopped

1 tsp. dried thyme

1 tsp. dried lemon thyme, if available

1 tsp. dried basil

1 tsp. dried marjoram

5 Chinese peppercorns (white pepper)

2 bay leaves

1 T. sea salt, or salt to taste

1 c. hulled barley

1 c. dry black-eyed peas

10-14 c. water

Place all ingredients except water in a 6-quart kettle or slow cooker. *Cover* with enough water to within 1/2 inch of the top, usually 10-14 cups. Cover. Bring to a *boil*. On stove top, turn down heat. In a slow cooker, leave on high. *Simmer* for at least 6 hours. Turn the slow cooker down to low. The longer this soup cooks, the better it is, although it is ready to eat after 6 hours. Be sure to check water level periodically. Serve hot.

Parsley, Sage, Rosemary and a Little More Soup

Cholesterol Free
Wheat/Gluten Free
Milk/Casein Free
Egg Free
Suitable through Stage IV

This is a good all year 'round soup that has a sweet and savory flavor. The black-eyed peas and peppercorns add some zing to the soup, while the potatoes give it great flavor. Started the soup the night before serving.

1 c. dried black-eyed peas

4 carrots, peeled and chopped

1/2 bunch celery, with leaves left on, chopped

4 red, firm potatoes, peeled and cubed

1 jar home-canned tomatoes, or 5 fresh tomatoes, chopped

2 bay leaves

8 peppercorns

1 T. sea salt + more to taste

1-1/2 tsp. dried rosemary, crushed between your fingers

1/2 tsp. dried sage

1/4 c. chopped fresh parsley

water to cover to within 1/2 inch of top of pot

Place all ingredients in a 6-quart slow cooker or kettle. *Cover*. If using the stove top method, bring to a boil, then reduce to *simmer* and cook for at least two hours, or until the beans are thoroughly cooked. If using the slow cooker, turn to "high" and cook several hours or overnight, then reduce to low to keep warm. Check water periodically, and add more if necessary. Serve hot.

Winter Comforts Soup

> *Cholesterol Free*
> *Milk/Casein Free*
> *Egg Free*
> *Suitable through Stage II*

A thick and hearty barley bean soup will drive out those winter chills. This soup takes a long time to reach its full flavor, so start early in the day or the night before.

2-3 "spring" onions (white bulb onions with greens) *or* 1 bunch scallions *or* 2 leeks, chopped

1 c. Great Northern or Navy beans

1 c. hulled barley

5-6 stalks and leaves of celery, chopped

sea salt to taste (2 tsp. to start)

10-14 c. water.

Place all ingredients into a 6-quart kettle or slow cooker. Add enough water to bring soup level within 1/2 inch of the top of the pot, usually about 10-14 cups. On the stovetop, cover, bring to boil, turn down to *simmer*. In a slow cooker, set on high, bring to a boil. *Cook* for at least 6 hours. Turn the slow cooker down to low after 6 hours. The longer this soup cooks, the better it is. Be sure to check water level periodically. This soup can be left in the slow cooker or on the stove top overnight, as long as there is adequate water. Check salt before serving. Enjoy.

Four Bean Soup

> *Cholesterol Free*
> *Wheat/Gluten Free*
> *Milk/Casein Free*
> *Egg Free*
> *Suitable through Stage IV*

This soup makes an exceptionally hearty meal. To serve at supper, start early in the day or even the night before. Serve as a main course, accompanied by **Herbed Brown Rice**, and a green salad topped with **Tomato Garlic Dressing**. Or, serve as a first course for any delicious meal. Serves 6-8 hungry people as a main course, or about 10 people as a first course.

1/2 c. dried garbanzo beans

1/2 c. dried brown lentils

1/2 c. dried navy beans

1/4 c. dried green split peas

1/2 c. short grain brown rice

1/2 c. red rice (sometimes called "Himalayan" rice)

2 T. fresh dill or 2 tsp. dried dill

4 tomatoes, chopped

3 medium potatoes, peeled and cubed

2 carrots, peeled and chopped

1 bunch scallions, chopped

4 stalks celery, chopped

1 tsp. celery seed

1 tsp. dill seed

1 tsp. dried basil

1 tsp. dried oregano

1 T. sea salt

9 c. water

Put all ingredients in a 6-quart slow cooker. Turn the heat on high, bring to a boil. Cook on high for at least 2-3 hours, then turn to medium heat and simmer until ready to serve. The longer this cooks, the better it tastes. This soup can cook up to 24 hours. Serve hot.

Sweet Pepper Soup

Cholesterol Free
Wheat/Gluten Free
Milk/Casein Free
Egg Free
Suitable through Stage IV

This soup has a very different, sweet flavor. Start early in the day or even the day before to bring out the full flavor.

    2 medium or 1 large leek, chopped

    2 c. chopped green beans

    2 sweet red bell peppers, chopped

    5 medium white potatoes, peeled and diced

    2 large tomatoes, chopped

    3 medium zucchini, sliced

    3 c. chopped celery

    1 c. dried garbanzo beans

    1 tsp. dried basil

    1 tsp. dried oregano

    1 tsp. dried dill

    1 T. sea salt

    10-14 c. water

Place all ingredients except water in a six quart slow cooker. Fill the slow cooker with water to within half and inch of the top, usually about 10-14 cups. Cover. Turn to high. Let cook several hours, then turn to low. Serve hot!

Hearty Barley, Bean and Onion Soup

Milk/Casein Free
Egg Free
Suitable through Stage II

This plain and hearty soup is great for winter.   The sweetness of the carrots and tomatoes is balanced by the sharpness of thyme and bay leaves. Be sure to start this soup early in the day or the night before serving, as it must simmer several hours to gain full flavor. You can cook it in a slow cooker while you are at work.

4 carrots, peeled and chopped

4 stalks celery, including leaves, chopped

2 fresh white onions with greens attached *or* 1 bunch scallions, chopped

4 fresh plum tomatoes, chopped

1 tsp. dried thyme

2 bay leaves

1 T. sea salt, or salt to taste

1/2 c. hulled barley

1/2 c. Great Northern beans

water

Place all ingredients in a 6-quart kettle or slow cooker. Cover with enough water to bring to within 1-1/2 inches of the top. Cover. Bring to a boil. If using stovetop, turn down to simmer. If using slow cooker, continue to cook at boil. Cook at least 6 hours before serving. The longer this soup cooks, the better it is. This soup can be left cooking overnight.   Be sure to check water level periodically. Serve hot.

Jade Soup

Cholesterol Free (using oil)
Wheat/Gluten Free
Milk/Casein Free (using oil)
Egg Free
Suitable through Stage IV

1 head cauliflower

1 bunch (10 oz.) fresh spinach *or* 1 package (10 oz.) frozen chopped spinach

2 T. butter or expeller pressed safflower oil

1 leek, chopped

4 medium turnips, peeled and diced

1 tsp. dried marjoram

1 tsp. dried basil

1 T. sea salt

8 peppercorns (optional)

10-14 c. water

Chop the white part of the cauliflower, including the tender parts of the stem, into bite sized pieces. *Prepare the spinach*: If using fresh spinach, wash it very thoroughly to remove all the sand. Chop into small pieces. If using frozen spinach, just open the package.   *Heat butter* or oil in a 6-quart kettle on medium heat. *Add* the leeks and saute for a few minutes, until soft. *Add* cauliflower, turnips and spinach. Cook a few minutes longer. Add the herbs, salt and peppercorns. Cover with water until within 1/2 inch of the top of the kettle. Bring to a boil, then reduce to simmer. Cook at least 2 to 6 hours. The longer you cook this, the more flavor it will have.

Lima Bean and Vegetable Soup

> *Cholesterol Free*
> *Wheat/Gluten Free*
> *Milk/Casein Free*
> *Egg Free*
> *Suitable through Stage IV*

Start this delicious soup early in the day or the night before for the best flavor.

2 T. or more expeller pressed safflower oil

2-3 white salad onions with green tops *or* 1 bunch scallions *or* 2 leeks, chopped

2 large carrots, peeled and chopped

2-4 parsnips, peeled and chopped

4 large celery stalks, including tops, chopped

3 large, firm red potatoes, peeled and cubed

1/2 c. dried baby lima beans

1/2 c. hulled barley or brown rice (use the brown rice for Wheat/Gluten Free soup)

1 T. sea salt or more to taste

1 tsp. dried thyme

1 tsp. dried dill

10-14 c. water

Heat 2 T. of oil in a 6-quart kettle. When the oil is hot, *add* the onions; saute a few minutes. Then add the carrots, parsnips and celery. *Saute* until the celery is soft. *Add* more oil if necessary to prevent sticking. When the celery is soft, add the potatoes, beans, barley or rice, herbs and salt. Add enough water to come within 1/2 inches of the top of the kettle, usually 10-14 cups. Cover. Bring to a boil; reduce to simmer. *Simmer* at least 3 hours, or until the beans are soft. The longer this cooks, the thicker it gets, and the better it tastes.

Chunky Autumn Vegetable Soup

> *Cholesterol Free*
> *Wheat/Gluten Free*
> *Milk/Casein Free*
> *Egg Free*
> *Suitable through Stage IV*

This soup is full of delicious fresh vegetables available at the turn of the season, and is great on those early dark evenings when the weather turns crisp. Start early in the day.

2 T. expeller pressed safflower oil

5 c. coarsely chopped broccoli

2 large or 3 medium zucchini, sliced

3 kohlrabi, peeled and diced

2 large or 4 medium russet potatoes, peeled and diced

3 carrots, peeled and chopped

2 large or 3 medium tomatoes, chopped

2 T. finely chopped Cubanel or other very mild chili pepper

water

1/2 tsp. dried thyme

1 tsp. dill seed

1 tsp. celery seed

1 T. sea salt, or salt to taste

10-14 c. water

In a 6-quart kettle, *heat the oil* until hot. *Add* the broccoli. While the broccoli is cooking, stir occasionally to prevent sticking. *Add* zucchini. *Add* kohlrabi and potatoes, then the carrots, tomatoes and pepper. When the vegetables begin to get soft, *add the herbs* salt. Mix through. Add enough water to come to within half an inch of the top of the kettle, usually 10-14 cups. Cover; bring to a boil; reduce to simmer. The soup is cooked when the vegetables are soft, but for greater flavor, cook for several hours to overnight.

Birthday Minestrone

> *Cholesterol Free (using oil)*
> *Wheat/Gluten Free*
> *Milk/Casein Free (using oil)*
> *Egg Free*
> *Suitable through Stage IV*

This soup was created in honor of our baby's first birthday, and is a real birthday treat. Start early in the day. This soup takes a minimum of four hours to cook after all the ingredients (except noodles) are in the pot.

2 T. expeller pressed safflower oil or butter

1 c. chopped celery

4 c. chopped broccoli

2 c. chopped green beans

4 medium zucchini, sliced

1 T. sea salt

1 tsp. dried dill

1 tsp. dried thyme

1 tsp. dried basil

1 tsp. dill seed

3 medium tomatoes, chopped

1 c. dried garbanzo beans (chick peas) or other mild beans

5 oz. (1/2 box) "Pastariso" brand rice spaghetti

water

In a six quart kettle, **melt the butter** or heat the oil, then **add** the celery. **Saute** a few minutes. Add the broccoli, continuing to saute. After a few minutes, add the green beans, zucchini, salt and herbs. After a few minutes, add the chopped tomatoes. Saute the vegetables until the celery is soft. Add the dried beans. Add enough water to come within a half inch of the top of the pot, approximately 10 cups. Add the salt. Cover; bring to a *boil*, then reduce to *simmer*. Cook for at least four hours. When the beans are soft, bring the soup to a boil again. Break the spaghetti into small pieces (1/2 inch to 1 inch long). Add to the soup. Reduce to simmer. Cook until the noodles are done, about 10 minutes. Mix thoroughly. Taste; add salt if needed. Serve soon after the noodles are done!

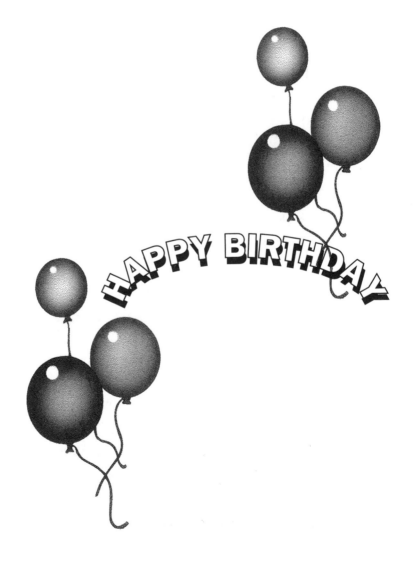

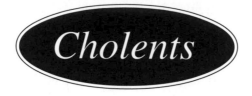

Rice Cholent

> *Cholesterol Free*
> *Wheat/Gluten Free*
> *Milk/Casein Free*
> *Egg Free*
> *Suitable through Stage IV*

"Cholent" is a traditional Eastern European Jewish dish, usually prepared for the Sabbath when cooking must be done in advance. Cholent recipes are as varied as the number of people in any community.   Start this recipe the night before serving.

3/4 c. dried garbanzo beans

3/4 c. any other dried beans except black beans Choose from: baby lima, small red, kidney, navy, lentils, pintos, etc.

2 c. brown rice

4 medium red potatoes, peeled and diced

3 tsp. sea salt

Optional seasonings: one pinch of each of rosemary and basil; *or* rosemary and tarragon; *or* oregano and basil (Italian style). Be creative!

water to come to within 1-1/2 inches of top of slow cooker

Butter at serving time (optional)

Place all ingredients in a slow cooker. Cook on high for at least 8 hours.   Turn the slow cooker to low until you serve. Check the cholent from time to time.   If you do not stir the cholent, a thick crust will form on top and bottom that some people love to eat. Serve plain or with a small amount of butter to add extra flavor.

Barley Cholent

Cholesterol Free
Milk/Casein Free
Egg Free
Suitable through Stage II

"Cholent" is a traditional Eastern European Jewish dish, usually prepared for the Sabbath when cooking must be done in advance. Cholent recipes are as varied as the number of people in any community.   Start cooking the night before serving.

3/4 c. dry garbanzo beans

3/4 c. other dry beans, except black beans. Choose from: baby lima, soy, small red, kidney, navy, lentils, pintos.

1 c. hulled barley

1 c. other grain. Choose from millet, rice, or wheat berries

3 tsp. sea salt

Optional seasonings: Good combinations include: rosemary and basil; rosemary and tarragon; oregano and basil (Italian style); curry, cumin and cardamon (Indian style). Be creative!

water to come to within 1-1/2 inches of the top of the slow cooker

Butter at serving time (optional)

Place all ingredients in a slow cooker. Add herbs as desired from combinations above. Use a pinch of each. *Cover* with ample water, about twice the amount of water as dry ingredients. Turn to high for at least 8 hours, then turn to low. Check the water occasionally.   If you do not stir the cholent, a thick crust will form on top and bottom that some people love to eat.   Serve plain or with a small amount of butter to add extra flavor

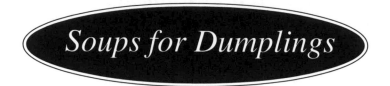

Tomato Vegetable Soup for Matzah Balls

Cholesterol Free
Wheat/Gluten Free
Milk/Casein Free
Egg Free
Suitable through Stage IV

This soup will make you wonder why you ever thought of chicken soup for matzah balls. The longer this cooks, the better it tastes. Start early in the day or the night before.

2 medium red potatoes, peeled and diced

4 carrots, chopped

1 quart home-canned tomatoes or 5 fresh tomatoes, peeled and chopped

4 zucchini, sliced

2 c. chopped green beans, chopped

3/4 c. navy beans, picked over and washed

2 T. salt

1 T. dried oregano

1 tsp. dried marjoram

1 tsp. dried thyme

1/8 tsp. black pepper (optional)

10-14 c. water

1 recipe *Matzah Balls* or *Rice & Dill Dumplings*

Place all of the ingredients except water into a 6-quart kettle or slow cooker. Cover with enough water to come to within 1/2 inch of the top. If using the stove top method, bring to a boil, then simmer for several hours, to overnight. If using a slow cooker, cook on the highest setting for several hours. When the beans are cooked, turn to low. Fully cook the soup before adding the dumplings. The longer the soup cooks, the better it tastes. Then add *Matzah Balls* or *Rice & Dill Dumplings* individually to each bowl just before serving. Serve hot.

Menu

for a Passover Seder

Haroset for Passover (p.119)

Gefilte Fish (p. 292)

Eggplant Tomato Relish (p.277)

Tomato Vegetable Soup for Matzah Balls (p. 142)

-or-

Vegetable Soup for Matzah Balls (p. 145)

Vegetarian Matzah Balls (p.144)

-or-

Rice & Dill Dumplings (p.146)

Green Salad with Lemon Herb Dressing (p.100)

Traditional or Light Potato Kugel (p.246-47)

Lemon Roasted Potatoes (p.244)

Vegetable Herb Souffle (p.270)

Roast Turkey with

Basil Rice Stuffing (p.242) (if permissible)

Carrot Tzimmes (p.278)

Raspberry Sorbet (p.350)

Passover Sponge Cake (p.320)

Vegetarian Matzah Balls

Milk/Casein Free
Suitable through Stage II

This recipe makes about 10 matzah balls. To make more, increase all of the ingredients proportionately except the eggs. For two recipes, use 7 eggs. For three recipes (enough to feed an army), use 10 eggs. Start early in the day to serve at supper time. Cooked matzah balls freeze well, so make plenty in advance, then defrost as needed. Serve with *Vegetable Soup for Matzah Balls* or *Tomato Vegetable Soup for Matzah Balls*.

  4 eggs

  2 T. butter, melted

  2 T. expeller pressed safflower oil

  1 tsp. sea salt

  1 c. matzah meal (white, whole wheat, or 1/2 and 1/2)

  water for boiling

Beat eggs, butter, oil and sea salt. *Mix in* matzah meal. Beat only enough to blend in. The more you beat the mixture, the harder the cooked matzah balls will be. *Cover and refrigerate* at least 30 minutes. *Boil* water in a large pot. When water is boiling, *quickly shape* the batter into small balls (about 1 inch diameter). My rule of thumb is no more than three turns to a ball. The less you handle the batter, the softer your matzah balls will be. Drop the balls into boiling water, and keep the water at a rapid boil for 20 minutes. Drain the water. To allow the matzah balls to absorb the flavor of the soup, take out a little of the broth from *Vegetarian Soup for Matzah Balls* or *Tomato Vegetable Soup for Matzah Balls* and place the broth in the pot with matzah balls. Serve matzah balls individually in each bowl with the rest of the soup. Spoon out and place in hot soup.

Vegetable Soup for Matzah Balls

Cholesterol Free (using oil)
Wheat/Gluten Free
Milk/Casein Free (using oil)
Egg Free
Suitable through Stage IV

This soup will change forever the idea that matzah balls need chicken soup!   The longer it cooks, the better it tastes. Make the soup separately from the *Matzah Balls*, then add the matzah balls or *Rice & Dill Dumplings*.

2 T. expeller pressed safflower oil plus a little more if necessary

2-3 white salad onions with green tops *or* 1 bunch scallions *or* 2 leeks, chopped

2 large carrots, peeled and chopped

2-4 parsnips, peeled and chopped

4 large celery stalks with tops, chopped

1 T. sea salt

dried herbs: 1/2 tsp. each basil, thyme and marjoram

16-18 c. water

One recipe of either *Matzah balls* or *Rice & Dill Dumplings*.

Heat oil in a 6-quart kettle on medium heat.   When the oil is hot, add the onions. *Saute* until soft. *Add* the celery, carrots and parsnips. *Saute* until the celery is soft. If necessary, add more oil to prevent sticking. Add the herbs and salt.   Add enough water to come within 1 inch of the top of the kettle, usually about 16-18 cups. *Cover*. Bring to a boil; reduce to a simmer. Cook several hours to overnight, if safe. Add *Matzah Balls* or *Rice & Dill Dumplings* individually to the bowls as you serve.

Rice & Dill Dumplings

Cholesterol Free
Wheat/Gluten Free
Milk/Casein Free
Egg Free
Suitable through Stage IV

These dumplings are fun to make, especially for kids. Serve plain, with butter and salt, or serve with *Vegetable Soup for Matzah Balls* or *Tomato Vegetable Soup for Matzah Balls*. This recipe makes about 20 balls.

12 c. water

2 c. Ener-G Rice Mix

1 tsp. sea salt

1 tsp. dried dill weed

4 T. expeller pressed safflower oil

1-2 c. water or less

water for cooking

Bring the water to a boil in a 4 to 6-quart pot. While the water is heating, combine the rice mix with the salt and dill. Add the oil. Mix well. Gradually add the water, mixing after each addition, until the dough holds a shape. Depending on the humidity, this may only require one cup. Form into small balls, about 1/2 inch to 1 inch in diameter. When the water is boiling vigorously, add the balls to the water. Cook at a rolling boil for 15 minutes. Do not overcook. The longer they cook, the more flour dissolves in the water. Deeelicious.

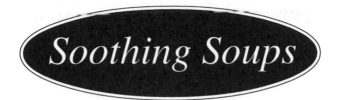

Celery 'N Thyme Soup

Cholesterol Free (using oil)
Wheat/Gluten Free
Milk/Casein Free (using oil)
Egg Free
Suitable through Stage IV

A nice comforting broth, especially in the winter. Great for those times when you need something warm and smooth.

2 T. expeller pressed safflower oil *or* butter

4 stalks celery, chopped

1/2 leek (optional), chopped

3 medium sized red potatoes, peeled and diced

1 tsp. dried thyme

1 large bay leaf

1/2 tsp. dried rosemary

1 tsp. sea salt, or more to taste

8-10 c. water

Heat the oil or butter in a 3-quart pot. When hot, *add* the celery, leek and potatoes. *Saute* until the vegetables are soft. *Add* the thyme, bay leaf, rosemary and salt. Add enough water to come within 1/2 inch of top of pot. Cover. *Bring to a boil*, turn to simmer and cook at least 2 hours. Adjust salt before serving.

Thick 'N Chunky Tomato Soup

Cholesterol Free
Wheat/Gluten Free
Milk/Casein Free
Egg Free
Suitable through Stage IV

This rich and chunky homemade tomato soup is just the thing for a cold winter day, or, served chilled, for a hot summer day. This tastes great with *Pizza Bread* and a green salad topped with *Lemon Herb Salad Dressing*.

12 large fresh tomatoes

3 large cloves garlic, chopped

1 tsp. sea salt

1 T. unprocessed clover honey

If time allows, *peel the tomatoes* by parboiling them for a few minutes, plunging in ice water and peeling. Not peeling them is OK, too, but the soup will not be as smooth. *Cut tomatoes* into chunks. Place them in a 4 or 6-quart pot. This recipe only makes 3-quarts, but the extra room for boiling is nice. *Add* the garlic. *Add* the salt and honey. *Slowly bring the soup* to a boil, on medium low heat. *Stir* to prevent scorching. *Cook* about 45 minutes. *Puree* about three fourths of the soup in a blender or with a hand puree tool designed for pureeing soups in the pot. If you do not like chunks, puree the entire batch. Serve hot or cold.

Italian Vegetable Soup

> *Cholesterol Free*
> *Wheat/Gluten Free*
> *Milk/Casein Free*
> *Egg Free*
> *Suitable through Stage IV*

This soup is an excellent all purpose clear soup. Serve it alone or with **Basic Brown Rice** or **Fluffy Rice**. Start this at least 4 hours before you plan to serve.

2 T. butter or expeller pressed safflower oil

4 stalks celery, chopped

4 small parsnips, peeled and chopped

3 medium zucchini, sliced

4 medium to large tomatoes, chopped

3 medium red potatoes, peeled and diced

2 tsp. dried basil

2 tsp. dried oregano

1 T. sea salt

10-14 c. water

Heat the oil or melt the butter in a 6-quart kettle on medium heat. *Add* the celery and *saute* until soft. *Add* the parsnips and zucchini. Continue sauteing until all vegetables are soft. Add the herbs, tomatoes and potatoes. Cook for a few minutes. Add salt. *Add the water* to within one half inch of the top of the kettle, usually 10-14 cups. Bring to a boil; simmer. Cook at least 3 hours. This soup tastes extra special when it cooks overnight.

Chili Dilly Soup

> *Cholesterol Free (using oil)*
> *Wheat/Gluten Free*
> *Milk/Casein Free*
> *Egg Free*
> *Suitable through Stage IV*

This is one of our favorite soups, all year round. It is very mild but with a hint of chili, juxtaposed against the fresh taste of dill and celery. This is a delicious way to start a meal. If you like a spicier soup, drop in a few cloves of garlic. Guests love this soup.

2 T. butter or expeller pressed safflower oil

3 medium zucchini, sliced

1-1/4 c. chopped or sliced celery

2 T. chopped fresh mild green chili peppers, such as Cubanel peppers

3 jumbo russet potatoes, peeled and cubed

1 T. sea salt

1 T. dried dill or 3 T. fresh dill

3 cloves garlic, chopped (optional)

10-14 c. water

Melt the butter or heat the oil in the bottom of a 6-quart kettle. When butter is hot, *add* the zucchini and celery. *Saute* until vegetables are soft. *Add* the chili pepper and continue sauteing. Add the potatoes, salt and dill. If you like a spicier soup, peel three cloves of garlic and just drop them in. *Fill* with water to reach to 1/2 inch of top of kettle, usually 10-14 cups. *Cover*; bring to a boil, reduce to simmer, and cook 1 hour.

Basic Vegetable Broth

Cholesterol Free
Wheat/Gluten Free
Milk/Casein Free
Egg Free
Suitable through Stage IV

Sometimes you just need a basic vegetable broth for those down in the dumps days. This is great for colds and flu, too. Add **Basic Brown Rice** or **Fluffy Rice** for a light meal.

2 T. expeller pressed safflower oil

3 large zucchini, sliced

1 large parsnip, peeled and chopped

3 large or 4 medium tomatoes, chopped

1 T. dried basil

1 T. dried oregano

1 T. sea salt

6-10 c. water

Heat the oil in a 3-quart pot on medium heat. When the oil is hot, **add** the zucchini and parsnips. **Saute** until soft. **Add** the tomatoes, herbs and salt. **Cover** with water to within one half inch of the top, usually 6-10 cups. Cover; **bring** to a boil; reduce to simmer. Cook for about 25 minutes, until vegetables are cooked through. Serve hot.

Beet Borscht

> *Cholesterol Free*
> *Wheat/Gluten Free*
> *Milk/Casein Free*
> *Egg Free*
> *Suitable through Stage IV*

For beet lovers only, this borscht is light and sweet. You can serve it hot or cold.

  5 beets

  1 tsp. dill seed

  1/2 tsp. sea salt, plus more to taste

  1 T. unprocessed clover honey

  water

Peel the beets and dice them into 1/2 inch cubes. *Place* them in a 3-quart saucepan with the other ingredients except water. *Fill* the pot with as much water as you need to come within 1/2 inch of the top of the pot. *Cover*; bring to a boil. Reduce to simmer. *Cook* at least 30 minutes, until the beets are soft. Serve hot or cold. If you eat dairy, serve with sour cream or plain yogurt.

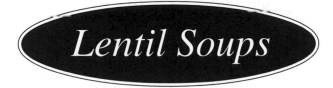

Celery Lentil Soup

Cholesterol Free (using oil)
Wheat/Gluten Free
Milk/Casein Free (using oil)
Egg Free
Suitable through Stage IV

This is a good old-fashioned lentil soup, with just a hint of spice.

2 T. butter or expeller pressed safflower oil

4 medium sized red tomatoes, chopped

3 c. coarsely chopped celery, including tops

2 tsp. dried marjoram

1 T. sea salt

1 tsp. dill seed

1/2 c. green or brown lentils

6-8 c. water

Melt the butter or heat the oil in a 3-quart pot. *Add* the celery and saute until soft. *Add* the marjoram, salt and dill seed. *Pick over* the lentils to discard obviously moldy ones. *Add* them to the other ingredients and mix. *Add water* to come to within 1/2 inch of the top of the pot, usually 6-8 cups. Cover; bring to a boil, reduce to simmer. Cook until lentils are soft, about 20 minutes.

Zucchini Lentil Soup

Cholesterol Free
Wheat/Gluten Free
Milk/Casein Free
Egg Free
Suitable through Stage IV

This soup is a favorite of family and friends. This soup can be served after only 30 minutes of cooking, but tastes best started early in the day and served for supper. If the soup gets very thick, you can add more water or serve it over **Basic Brown Rice** for a delicious main dish.

2 T. expeller pressed safflower oil

2 leeks (optional), chopped

4 medium zucchini, sliced

3 c. green or brown lentils

1 T. dried basil

2 large tomatoes, chopped

1 T. dried dill or 4 T. fresh dill

2 T. sea salt, or salt to taste

14-16 c. water

2 additional tomatoes (optional), chopped

4 scallions (optional), chopped

Heat the oil in a 6-quart kettle. *Add* the leeks; saute until soft. Then *add* the zucchini. Cook until soft.   Then pick over the lentils for obviously moldy ones and rinse. Add the lentils to the zucchini-leek mixture. Saute for a minute or so. Add the 2 chopped tomatoes. Add the herbs and salt. *Fill the kettle* with enough water to come within 1/2 inch of the top of the kettle, approximately 14-16 cups. Cover. *Bring to a boil*, then reduce to a simmer for at least 30 minutes, until lentils are cooked. This tastes best when simmered for several hours. Just before serving, garnish with additional chopped tomatoes and scallions.

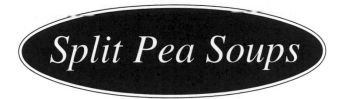

Our Favorite Split Pea Soup

Cholesterol Free (using oil)
Wheat/Gluten Free
Milk/Casein Free (using oil)
Egg Free
Suitable through Stage IV

Of all the split pea soups, this has become our favorite. It has the full flavor of split peas without the heaviness of traditional split pea soup. Everyone who eats this loves it, even people who swear they can't stand split pea soup! Serve piping hot with *Delicious and Nutritious Whole Wheat Bread*, or *Fluffy Rice*, and a green salad topped with *Lemon Herb Salad Dressing*.

   2 T. butter or expeller pressed safflower oil

   5-6 stalks celery, chopped into one-inch lengths

   4 medium red potatoes, peeled and cubed into half inch cubes

   1/2 c. dried navy beans

   2 c. dried green split peas

   2 tsp. dried marjoram

   1 tsp. dried dill

   1 T. sea salt

   12-14 c. water

Heat the butter or oil in a 6-quart kettle. Add the celery and *saute* until soft. *Add* the potatoes, navy beans, split peas, herbs and salt. Add water to within one half inch of the top of the pot, usually 12-14 cups. Cover. Bring to a boil; reduce to simmer. Cook at least 3 hours, until navy beans are soft.

Celery Soup with a Hint of Splits

> *Cholesterol Free (using oil)*
> *Wheat/Gluten Free*
> *Milk/Casein Free*
> *Egg Free*
> *Suitable through Stage IV*

This soup is a compromise between those who love split peas and those who would prefer never to see split peas served on their table. The soup is very light and has the slightest hint of the split pea flavor.

2 T. butter or expeller pressed safflower oil

6-7 stalks celery, including tops, chopped

4 medium sized red tomatoes, peeled and diced

2 tsp. dried marjoram

1 T. sea salt

1 tsp. dill seed

1/2 c. split peas

water

Heat the oil or butter, or a combination of the two, in a 3-quart pot. When the oil is hot or the butter melted, *add the celery* and saute until soft. *Add* the rest of the ingredients. Add water to come to within 1/2 inch of top of pot. *Cover*; bring to a boil, reduce to simmer. *Cook* until peas are soft, about 20 minutes.

Split Pea Soup for Pea Lovers Only

Cholesterol Free
Wheat/Gluten Free
Milk/Casein Free
Egg Free
Suitable through Stage IV

This is a favorite winter dish, hearty enough for the main course. If you love split pea soup, you'll make this again and again. Start this soup at least 4 hours before serving.

2-3 T. expeller pressed safflower oil

4 large stalks celery, including tops, chopped

2 carrots, peeled and chopped

2-3 green-topped white onions *or* 1 bunch scallions *or* 2 leeks, chopped

3 large red potatoes, peeled and diced

3 c. green split peas

1 bay leaf

1 tsp. dried thyme

1 tsp. dried basil

1 T. sea salt (or to taste)

10-14 c. water

Heat enough safflower oil in a 6-quart kettle to cover the bottom in a thin layer, usually about 2-3 tablespoons. *Add* the celery, carrots, and onions. *Saute* until soft. Add the potatoes. *Saute a few minutes*, then add split peas, herbs and salt, and enough water to come to about 1 inch from the top of a 6-quart kettle, usually about 10-14 cups. *Cover;* bring to boil; reduce to simmer. Cook at least 4 hours.   Check the water level periodically.   Check seasonings and adjust if necessary before serving.

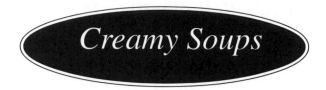

Creamy Soups

Cream of Zucchini Soup

Cholesterol Free (using oil)
Wheat/Gluten Free
Milk/Casein Free
Egg Free
Suitable through Stage IV

This is a favorite summer soup. It can be served warm or cold, so advance preparation is easy.

2 T. butter or 2 T. expeller pressed safflower oil

2 leeks (optional), chopped

6 medium zucchini, sliced

6 large red potatoes (more for a thicker soup, fewer for a thinner soup), peeled and diced

1 T. dried basil

1/2 T.dried marjoram

1/2 T. dried thyme

2 T. sea salt, or salt to taste

12-14 c. water

Heat the butter or oil in a 6-quart kettle. When the butter is melted or the oil is hot, *add* the leeks and saute until soft. *Add* the zucchini. When the zucchini is bright, add the herbs and salt. Add the potatoes. *Add enough water* to come within 1/2 inch of the top, usually 12-14 cups. *Cover*. Bring to a boil, then simmer for at least 30 minutes, until all of the vegetables are cooked. *Cool* to a manageable temperature. *Puree* the soup in a blender or with a hand mixer designed for pureeing soups in the pot. Make the soup very smooth. You're ready to serve, hot or cold.

Cream of Broccoli Soup

Cholesterol Free (using oil)
Wheat/Gluten Free
Milk/Casein Free
Egg Free
Suitable through Stage IV

Broccoli is plentiful and fresh in the late summer and fall, so take advantage! This soup can be served warm or cold, so advance preparation is easy.

2 T. butter or 2 T. expeller pressed safflower oil

2 leeks, chopped

1 large bunch of broccoli, chopped

1 T. dried basil

1/2 T. dried marjoram

1/2 T. dried thyme

2 T. sea salt, or salt to taste

6 large red potatoes (more for a thicker soup, fewer for a thinner soup), peeled and diced

Heat the butter or oil in a 6-quart kettle. When the butter is melted or the oil is hot, *add* the leeks and saute until soft. *Add* the broccoli. When the broccoli is bright, add the herbs and salt. Add the potatoes. *Add enough water* to come within 1/2 inch of the top, usually 12-14 cups. *Cover.* Bring to a boil, then *simmer* for at least 30 minutes, until all of the vegetables are cooked. *Cool* to a manageable temperature. *Puree* the soup in a blender or with a hand mixer designed for pureeing soups in the pot. Make the soup very smooth. You're ready to serve, hot or cold.

Cream of Zucchini and Broccoli Soup

Cholesterol Free (using oil)
Wheat/Gluten Free
Milk/Casein Free
Egg Free
Suitable through Stage IV

This summer soup is lighter than broccoli soup but heartier than zucchini soup. It can be served warm or cold, so advance preparation is easy.

2 T. butter or 2 T. expeller pressed safflower oil

l large bunch broccoli, chopped

4 medium zucchini, sliced

1 T. dried basil

1/2 T. dried marjoram

1/2 T. dried thyme

2 T. sea salt, or salt to taste

6 large red potatoes (more for a thicker soup, fewer for a thinner soup), peeled and diced

12-14 c. water

Heat the butter or oil in a 6-quart kettle. *Add the broccoli* and zucchini. Saute. When the vegetables are bright, add the herbs and salt . Cook for a few minutes, then add the potatoes. *Add* enough water to come within 1/2 inch of the top, usually 12-14 cups. Cover. *Bring to a boil*, then simmer at least 30 minutes. *Cool* to a manageable temperature. *Puree* the soup in a blender or with a hand mixer designed for pureeing soups in the pot. Make the soup very smooth. You're ready to serve! This soup is also excellent cold, so place in the refrigerator and serve the next day.

Cream of Pizza Soup

> *Cholesterol Free (using oil)*
> *Wheat/Gluten Free*
> *Milk/Casein Free*
> *Egg Free*
> *Suitable through Stage IV*

A white soup that uses no tomatoes, has no cheese and no bread—called pizza soup? Just try it. You'll love it. Created by our daughter, we find that children ask for this soup again and again.

1 T. butter or expeller pressed safflower oil

1 large leek (optional), chopped

2 cloves garlic, chopped

7 red potatoes plus more for a thicker soup, peeled and diced

1 T. sea salt

1 tsp. dried basil

1 tsp. dried oregano

1/8 tsp. dried dill

8-10 c. water, plus more to taste

Heat the butter or oil in a 3-quart saucepan. When the oil or butter is hot, *add* the leeks and garlic. *Saute* until soft. *Add* the potatoes. Continue sauteing for a few minutes. *Add* the salt and herbs. *Add water* to within 1/2 inch of the top of the saucepan, approximately 8-10 cups. Cover. *Bring to a boil*, then reduce to simmer for 20-30 minutes. When the potatoes are very soft, cool to a manageable temperature. *Puree* the soup in a blender or with a hand blender designed for pureeing soups. Make sure you puree long enough to get a smooth consistency. This has a nice, smooth consistency—not too thick, not too thin, and tastes like a creamy pizza. For a thicker soup, use more potatoes. Serve hot!

Cream of Asparagus Soup

Cholesterol Free (using oil)
Wheat/Gluten Free
Milk/Casein Free
Egg Free
Suitable through Stage IV

Asparagus is a great treat when in season. This soup takes full advantage of those precious weeks. Like the other cream soups, you can serve this one hot or cold.

2 lbs. asparagus

6 large red potatoes (more for a thicker soup, fewer for a thinner soup)

2 T. butter or 2 T. expeller pressed safflower oil for sauteing

1 T. dried basil

1/2 T. dried marjoram

1/2 T. dried thyme

2 T. sea salt, or salt to taste

12-14 c. water

Cut off the tough ends of the asparagus, then *chop* into 1-2 inch lengths. *Peel and chop* the potatoes. *Heat the oil* or butter in a 6-quart pot. When the butter is melted or the oil is hot, *add* the asparagus and *saute* until bright. *Add the herbs* and potatoes. *Cover* the mixture with enough water to come within 1/2 inch of the top, usually 12-14 cups. Cover. *Bring to a boil*, then simmer until the potatoes are cooked, usually about 30 minutes. *Cool* to a manageable temperature. *Puree* the soup in a blender or with a hand mixer designed for pureeing soups in the pot. Make the soup very smooth. You're ready to serve! This soup is also excellent cold, so place in the refrigerator and serve the next day.

Creamy Harvest Soup

Cholesterol Free
Wheat/Gluten Free
Milk/Casein Free
Egg Free
Suitable through Stage IV

A nice, smooth soup for those rainy Fall days, made with nothing but vegetables, water and salt, but oh so good. This soup has a nice mild flavor and a light orange color. The recipe makes about 5 quarts. If you are dining alone, or cooking for just two people, either halve the recipe or freeze the leftovers.

4 medium sized red potatoes, peeled and cubed

4 medium sized kohlrabi, peeled and cubed

4 medium sized parsnips, peeled and chopped

4 medium sized turnips, peeled and chopped

6 carrots, peeled and chopped

4 stalks celery, tops included, chopped

2 T. sea salt

10-14 c. water

butter (optional-use only if not watching dairy or cholesterol intake)

Combine all of the ingredients into a 6-quart kettle. Bring to a *boil*; cover; simmer for about two hours. When the vegetables are thoroughly cooked and soft, *cool* to a manageable temperature. *Puree* the soup in a blender on high speed, or use a tool that will puree the soup in the pot. Make sure the soup is well-pureed. It should not be mealy or grainy. If desired, add small amounts of butter to the pot or to individual servings. Serve hot.

Cream of Spinach Soup

> *Cholesterol Free (using oil)*
> *Wheat/Gluten Free*
> *Milk/Casein Free*
> *Egg Free*
> *Suitable through Stage IV*

This cream of spinach soup is a surprising light and fresh alternative to traditionally heavy cream of spinach soups.

4 white rose or red potatoes, peeled and cubed

1 large leek, chopped

2 large cloves garlic, chopped

1 tsp. dried basil or 1 T. fresh chopped basil

2 tsp. sea salt

4 c. water

10 oz. fresh spinach, or, if unavailable1- 10 oz. package frozen chopped spinach

2 T. butter or expeller pressed safflower oil

Place the potatoes, leek and garlic in a 3-quart saucepan with the basil, 1 tsp. salt, and water.   Cover; bring to a boil, then reduce to simmer. *Cook* for about 20-30 minutes, or until potatoes are soft enough to mash. While the potatoes are cooking, thoroughly *wash* the spinach, leaf by leaf, so no sand or dirt remains. *Chop* finely. If you are using frozen spinach, defrost it and squeeze the water out. *Melt* the butter or heat the oil in a frying pan. *Add* the spinach. *Sprinkle* with 1 teaspoonful salt. *Saute* until the spinach is just cooked and still bright green. *Remove* from the heat and set aside. When potatoes are cooked, *cool* to a manageable temperature. Then *puree* the potato mixture in a blender or a hand blender that can puree foods in the cooking pot. Add the spinach mixture. Heat through and serve.

Cool Cream of Cucumber Soup

> *Cholesterol Free (without butter)*
> *Wheat/Gluten Free*
> *Milk/Casein Free*
> *Egg Free*
> *Suitable through Stage IV*

Cooked cucumbers give this soup a fresh and different taste than many other vegetable soups. This is perfect for a hot summer day.

7 large cucumbers

2 T. or more dried chervil *or* 1 T. dried chervil and 1 T. dried dill . If chervil is unavailable, use 2 T. dried dill instead

water

6 medium red potatoes (more for a thicker soup; fewer for a thinner soup)

2 T. butter (optional)

sea salt to taste

Peel the cucumbers. Make sure they are not bitter. Cut the cucumbers into large chunks. *Place in a saucepan* with the chervil and/or dill and with about a cup of water, enough to keep them from scorching. *Steam* the cucumbers until they are very soft. Remove from heat; *cool*. While the cucumbers are cooking, *peel and chop* the potatoes. Place the potato chunks into a pot separate from the cucumbers, with enough water to cover them. Bring them to a *boil*; lower heat and *simmer* until potatoes are very soft. *Cool* until you can handle the mixture safely. *Puree* the cucumbers and potatoes together, with their cooking water. Add salt to taste. Add butter, if desired. Serve hot or cold.

Cream of Cauliflower Soup

Cholesterol Free (using oil)
Wheat/Gluten Free
Milk/Casein Free
Egg Free
Suitable through Stage IV

For the cauliflower lovers only—this soup is deeelicious. It has the creamy consistency of the cheesy type of cauliflower soups, without the heaviness.

5 T. butter or expeller pressed safflower oil

1 head cauliflower (medium to large size)

2 T. chopped Cubanel or other very mild chili pepper (optional)

7 medium red potatoes, peeled and cubed

1 T. sea salt, or salt to taste

14 c. water, approximately

In a 6-quart kettle, *heat* the butter or oil. While the butter or oil is heating, *chop the cauliflower* into small pieces no more than two inches in diameter. Use the white part of the stems, but not the leaves. *Add* the cauliflower and the pepper. *Saute* until the cauliflower is soft and starts to turn golden brown. *Add* the potatoes and the salt. *Add enough water* to come within 1/2 inch of the top of the pot, approximately 14 cups. *Cover*; bring the soup to a boil; turn down to simmer. *Simmer* about 30 minutes until you can pierce the potatoes easily with a fork. *Cool* to a manageable temperature. *Puree* in a blender or with a hand blender designed to puree soups in the pot. Make sure you leave no lumps. *Heat* through and serve.

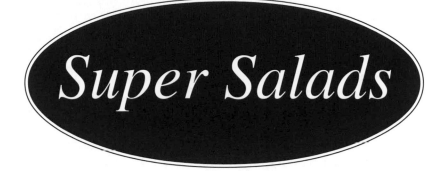

Super Salads

Salads can be served any time, and are the perfect food for sharing. Here you will find recipes for rice salads, potato salads and vegetable salads. Look in **Dressings and Sauces** *for more salad dressings.*

Mediterranean Rice Tabouli

Cholesterol Free
Wheat/Gluten Free
Milk/Casein Free
Egg Free
Suitable through Stage IV

Tabouli is a middle eastern salad usually made with bulgur, a type of cracked wheat. Characteristic of Tabouli is parsley, and lots of it! Using rice gives the salad a completely different appeal, light, tasty and filling. It is easy to make and should be made in advance This dish is especially good to bring to potlucks. Be sure to allow sufficient time to cool the cooked rice.

2-1/2 c. raw brown rice

7 c. water

2 cloves garlic

1/2 c. freshly squeezed lemon juice (about 4 lemons)

1/2 c. expeller pressed safflower oil

2 tsp. salt

1 lg. or two medium tomatoes

2 cucumbers (optional)

1-2 bunches fresh parsley

Combine the rice and water in a 3 quart pot. Cover. Bring to boil, then turn down to simmer. *Cook* until rice is tender. The rice will be firm. *Cool* completely. Set aside. *Peel the garlic* cloves and microwave for 20 seconds on high. *Chop* finely. *Add* to the rice. *Add* the lemon juice, safflower oil, and salt . *Mix* well. *Chop* the tomatoes and cucumbers into small pieces. *Chop* parsley very fine. *Add* these vegetables to the rice mixture. Mix well and chill!

Mediterranean Rice and Vegetable Salad

Cholesterol Free
Wheat/Gluten Free
Milk/Casein Free
Egg Free
Suitable through Stage IV

This salad can't be beat for flavor and color. You should start early in the day, or the night before. This salad is similar to **Mediterranean Rice Tabouli**, but uses no parsley and adds beans and other vegetables. This makes about 4 quarts of salad, and is great to take to potlucks.

4 cloves garlic

7 c. cooked brown rice

1 c. dried garbanzo beans, cooked according to directions in **Mainly Beans**

1/2 c. expeller pressed safflower oil

1/2 c. freshly squeezed lemon juice

1-1/2 tsp. sea salt

4 tomatoes, chopped

1 cucumber, peeled and chopped

1 red bell pepper, peeled and chopped

Peel the garlic and microwave on high for 20 seconds, then chop. Combine all ingredients in a large bowl. Mix well. Cover and refrigerate 2 hours to overnight.

Egg Salad

> *Milk/Casein Free*
> *Wheat/Gluten Free*
> *Suitable through Stage III*

Our guests love this egg salad. It has the full egg flavor, without the heaviness of mayonnaise. For a new variation, try using a little **Hummus** in place of some of the oil. For an entire meal, serve with one of or more of the other salads in this chapter, any of the soups, and **Basic Brown Rice**. Or, make a sandwich with **Delicious and Nutritious Whole Wheat Bread** . . .or, spread some egg salad on a rice cake and top with a tomato.

12 large or jumbo eggs

1 tsp. sea salt

4 T. expeller pressed safflower oil, plus more to taste

water as needed for desired consistency

2-3 stalks celery (optional)

Boil the eggs for 10-12 minutes, until hard boiled. **Cool** in cold water. When the eggs are cool enough to handle, **peel and mash** them. Mix in the salt. Add the oil. **Add a combination** of more oil and water until the salad is the desired consistency. If using the celery, **chop** the stalks into small pieces. **Add** to the eggs and mix. Refrigerate until ready to serve.

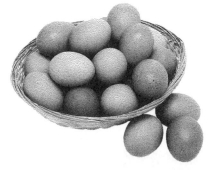

Spicy Egg Salad

Milk/Casein Free
Wheat/Gluten Free
Suitable through Stage III

This nontraditional egg salad is light and spicy. Serve it with other salads, such as **Basil Potato Salad**, a green salad with **Creamy Cucumber Dressing**, some **Basic Brown Rice** and any of our soups for a complete meal for 6-8 people.

12 large or jumbo eggs

1 tsp. sea salt

1/4 tsp. curry powder

1/4 tsp. dry yellow mustard

1/8 tsp. pepper

1/2 tsp. paprika

1/4 c. chopped scallions

4 T. expeller pressed safflower oil , plus more to taste

water for desired consistency

2-3 stalks celery (optional)

Boil the eggs for 10-12 minutes, until hard boiled. **Cool** in cold water. When cool enough to handle, **peel and mash** them. **Mix** in the salt, spices and scallions. **Add** the oil. Add a combination of more oil and water until the salad is the desired consistency. If using the celery, **chop the stalks** into small pieces and add to the egg salad. **Mix**. Refrigerate until ready to serve.

Parsley Potato Salad

> *Cholesterol Free*
> *Wheat/Gluten Free*
> *Milk/Casein Free*
> *Egg Free*
> *Suitable through Stage IV*

This recipe is a very light and delicious potato salad, another of our guests' favorites. Allow enough time to boil the potatoes and cool them fully before putting the salad together, then put the salad together at least a few hours before serving. This is a great "make ahead" dish for the next day's lunch or dinner. It's also a great potluck dish.

8 large red potatoes

water for boiling

water for cooling

1/4 c. chopped, fresh parsley

2 T. chopped fresh dill weed (optional)

1 tsp. sea salt

2 large tomatoes (optional)

approximately 6 tsp. expeller pressed safflower oil

Boil the potatoes, whole. When done, *pour* off the cooking water. *Cover* with fresh cold water. *Refrigerate* until cold. Cooling overnight is fine. Take the potatoes out and *peel* them by slipping off their skins. If the skins are hard to slip off, peel them under hot water. *Cut* potatoes into bite-sized cubes or chunks. Put potatoes in a large bowl. *Add* the chopped parsley, dill and salt. *Mix* thoroughly. For a different look, chop the two tomatoes and gently fold them in. Add 1 tsp. of oil for each approximate cup of potatoes you have in the bowl. Mix well. This is enough oil to provide a light coating. Refrigerate, covered, until ready to serve.

Dilled Potato Salad

Cholesterol Free
Wheat/Gluten Free
Milk/Casein Free
Egg Free
Suitable through Stage IV

This cool, refreshing potato salad is another favorite. Make this ahead to allow plenty of time for the dill to flavor the potatoes. This makes about 4 quarts of salad, enough to serve lots of hungry people.

8 large red potatoes

water for boiling

water for cooling

1/4 c. fresh chopped dill, or 2 tsp. dried dill

1 tsp. sea salt

approximately 6 tsp. expeller pressed safflower oil

Boil the potatoes, whole. When done, *drain* off the cooking water. *Cover* with fresh cold water. *Refrigerate* until cold. Cooling overnight is fine. Take the potatoes out and *peel them* by slipping off their skins. If the potatoes are hard to peel, put them under hot water. *Cut* potatoes into bite-sized cubes or chunks. Put potatoes in a large bowl. *Add* the dill. Mix well. *Sprinkle in* the salt while stirring. Add small amounts of salt at a time until all the salt is in. If you add all the salt at once, it will clump up. *Mix* thoroughly. *Add* 1 tsp. of oil for each approximate cup of potatoes you have in the bowl. *Mix well*. This is enough oil to provide a light coating. Refrigerate until ready to serve.

Asparagus Potato Salad

> *Cholesterol Free*
> *Wheat/Gluten Free*
> *Milk/Casein Free*
> *Egg Free*
> *Suitable through Stage IV*

This salad is a treat during asparagus season. Despite the detailed directions, this salad is very easy to prepare. Allow enough time to boil the potatoes and cool fully before putting the salad together.

> 8 large red potatoes
>
> water for cooking
>
> water for cooling
>
> 1 lb. fresh asparagus
>
> water for steaming
>
> 12 ice cubes
>
> water for cooling
>
> 1 tsp. sea salt
>
> approximately 6 tsp. expeller pressed safflower oil

Boil the potatoes, whole. When done, *pour* off the cooking water. *Cover* with fresh cold water. *Refrigerate* until cold. Cooling overnight is fine. While the potatoes are cooling, shortly before you peel them, *blanch the asparagus as follows:* First, *chop* the asparagus into one-inch pieces, discarding the tough ends. *Place* the pieces in a pan with about 1/4 to 1/2 inch of water. *Cook* on the stove top or in the microwave until the asparagus is just tender, not overcooked. *While the asparagus is cooking*, place cold water and ice cubes in a large bowl. As soon as the asparagus is cooked, *remove* from heat; *pour off* the hot water.

Plunge the asparagus into ice water and set aside. Now *peel the potatoes* by slipping off their skins. If the skins are hard to slip off, peel them under hot water. *Cut potatoes* into bite-sized cubes or chunks and put in a 4-quart serving bowl. *Add* the asparagus and salt. *Mix* thoroughly. *Add* 1 tsp. of oil for each approximate cup of potatoes you have in the bowl. *Mix* well. This is enough oil to provide a light coating. Refrigerate until ready to serve.

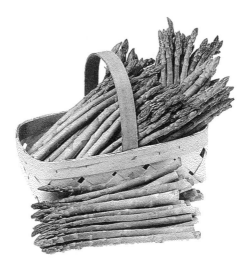

Bright and Sprightly Potato Vegetable Salad

> *Cholesterol Free*
> *Wheat/Gluten Free*
> *Milk/Casein Free*
> *Egg Free*
> *Suitable through Stage IV*

A basic potato salad becomes a work of art when perked up by the beautiful colors and flavors of fresh peppers, tomatoes and other vegetables. Allow enough time to boil the potatoes and cool fully before putting the salad together. This beautiful potluck dish is best when made ahead of time.

8 large red potatoes

water for cooking and for cooling

1/4 c. chopped, fresh parsley

1 tsp. sea salt

1 large, firm, sweet red bell pepper

1 large, firm, sweet green bell pepper

1 cucumber (optional), peeled and chopped into bite-sized pieces

approximately 6 tsp. expeller pressed safflower oil

Boil the potatoes, whole. When done, *pour* off the cooking water. *Cover* with fresh cold water. *Refrigerate* until cold. Cooling overnight is fine. *Peel the potatoes* by slipping off their skins. If the skins are hard to slip off, peel them under hot water. *Cut* potatoes into bite-sized cubes or chunks and place in a four-quart serving bowl. *Add* the chopped parsley and the salt. Mix thoroughly. *Seed and chop* the peppers into bite-sized pieces. Add to the salad. Add cucumbers. *Add* 1 tsp. of oil for each approximate cup of vegetables you have in the bowl. *Mix* well. *Refrigerate* until ready to serve.

Basil and Tomato Potato Salad

> Cholesterol Free
> Wheat/Gluten Free
> Milk/Casein Free
> Egg Free
> Suitable through Stage IV

This is a quintessential summer salad, when fresh basil and tomatoes are at their peak. Prepare this salad several hours before serving to allow the taste of the fresh basil to flavor the potatoes. This also is a great potluck dish. Makes about 4 quarts of potato salad.

8 large red potatoes

water for boiling

water for cooling

2 T. fresh, chopped basil, or 1 tsp. dried basil, plus more to taste

1 tsp. sea salt

1 large or 2 small fresh tomatoes, chopped

approximately 6 tsp. expeller pressed safflower oil

Boil the whole potatoes. When done, *pour* off the cooking water. Cover with fresh cold water. *Refrigerate* until cold. Cooling overnight is fine. *Peel the potatoes* by slipping off their skins. If peeling is difficult, peel them under hot water. *Cut potatoes* into bite-sized cubes or chunks. *Add the basil* and the salt. If you are adore basil, add more. *Mix thoroughly*. *Gently add* the tomatoes, being careful not to mash them. *Add* 1 tsp. of oil for each approximate cup of potatoes you have in the bowl. Mix well. This is enough oil to provide a light coating. Refrigerate until ready to serve.

Pasta Salad

> *Cholesterol Free*
> *Wheat/Gluten Free*
> *Milk/Casein Free*
> *Egg Free*
> *Suitable through Stage IV*

Pasta salad makes a great addition to any summer luncheon. Allow a few hours to cool the salad before serving to let the full flavor of the herbs come through. This makes about 4 quarts of salad, enough for a hungry family plus some guests. If you have fewer mouths to feed, cut the recipe in half.

2 pkg. (20 oz.) Pastariso brand rice spaghetti, vermicelli or fettucine *or*, if gluten is tolerated, 20 oz. whole wheat spaghetti, vermicelli or fettucine

small amount of expeller pressed safflower oil

1 tsp. sea salt

2 T. fresh basil

1 tsp. dried basil

1 tsp. dried oregano

4 medium tomatoes

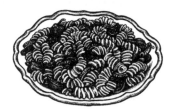

1/2 c. expeller pressed safflower oil

Optional: raw fresh vegetables, such as green beans, broccoli, zucchini

Cook the pasta according to package directions. **Drain, then** place in a four-quart serving bowl and **mix** with a small amount of oil to prevent sticking. **Refrigerate**. When the noodles are cold, **add** the rest of the oil. **Mix**. **Chop** the fresh basil and add it to the salad, along with the dried basil, oregano and salt. **Mix**. **Chop** the tomatoes and any other fresh vegetables into very small pieces. Mix them into the pasta well. Chill thoroughly before serving.

Simply Scrumptious Green and Red Salad

Cholesterol Free
Wheat/Gluten Free
Milk/Casein Free
Egg Free
Suitable through Stage IV

A few simple ingredients make this tantalizing salad special.
Take it to a potluck, or to serve it with your own luncheon.
Prepare this salad several hours before serving.

12 ice cubes

water

1 lb. fresh green beans

water for steaming

1 red bell pepper

1/4 c. freshly squeezed lemon juice

1/4 tsp. salt (optional)

Prepare a large bowl of ice water using at least a dozen ice cubes
and cold water. Set aside. *Cut off the ends* of the green beans, but
leave the beans long. Bring a small amount of water to a boil in a
saucepan and add the beans. *Steam* the beans just until tender, but
barely cooked. *Remove* the pan from the heat. *Immediately*
drain off the hot water, then *plunge* the beans into the bowl of ice
water. While the beans are cooling, *slice* the red pepper into very
thin strips. Set aside. When the beans are cold, drain them. *Mix*
the beans, peppers, lemon juice and salt (optional). Place in a
serving bowl, cover, and refrigerate for several hours or
overnight.

Cole Slaw

Cholesterol Free
Wheat/Gluten Free
Milk/Casein Free
Egg Free
Suitable through Stage IV

A cool, crisp cole slaw with lots of flavor makes a picnic great.
You should make this salad ahead to allow the flavors to mingle.

6 c. shredded or chopped green or Napa (Chinese) cabbage

3/4 c. shredded carrots

2 tsp. celery seed

1 tsp. sea salt

1/4 c. freshly squeezed lemon juice

For wilted cole slaw: place the shredded cabbage in a large
microwavable bowl, cover with plastic wrap and microwave for
30-60 seconds on high. *For crisp cole slaw*: use raw shredded
cabbage. *Continue for both cole slaws:* Mix cabbage, carrots,
lemon juice and seasonings together. Refrigerate several hours to
overnight. Serve cold. Makes about 4 cups of salad.

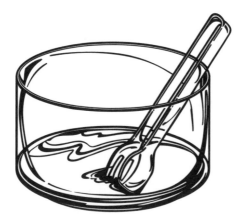

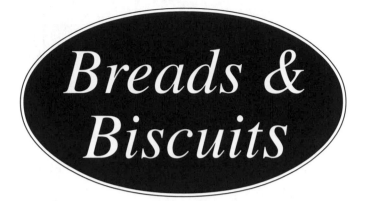

Bread has been called the staff of life. Even on a yeast free diet, you can enjoy:

       ~ *Breads*

       ~ *Biscuits*

       ~ *Pancakes*

       ~ *Muffins*

Delicious and Nutritious Whole Wheat Bread

Cholesterol Free
Milk/Casein Free
Egg Free
Suitable through Stage II

This tasty, cake-like bread is a favorite of everyone who tries it—even kids, who think it's cake. This bread is crumbly, so make sandwiches cautiously. This recipe makes two loaves. Double the recipe for extra bread. Freeze extra bread for later.

  expeller pressed safflower oil for greasing pans

  extra whole wheat flour for flouring pans

  1-1/2 c. old fashioned rolled oats

  2-1/2 c. water

  1/2 c. expeller pressed safflower oil

  1/2 c. unprocessed clover honey

  3 c. whole wheat flour or whole wheat pastry flour to start

  3 tsp. baking powder

  1/4 tsp. baking soda

  1 tsp. sea salt

  1-7 c. additional whole wheat flour or whole wheat pastry flour

  1 egg, beaten, for crust (optional)

  additional expeller-pressed safflower oil for crust.

1. Preheat the oven to 350F.

2. If using loaf pans, oil them well and flour them. If using cookie sheets, flour them. Set aside.

3. In a very large bowl, mix the oats, water, safflower oil, and

honey. Let this mixture sit for a few minutes. While the wet mixture is sitting, combine dry ingredients in another bowl (3 c. flour, baking powder, baking soda, and salt). Mix thoroughly. When oats are soft, add dry ingredients to wet. Stir well with a wooden spoon.

4. Add one cup of additional flour at a time, enough to make the dough manageable for mixing. You are ready to knead when the dough is very heavy, and pulls away from the sides of the bowl as you mix it. The dough should be the consistency of thick clay, but a little sticky. Your hands will get very sticky kneading the dough, but just enjoy the experience!

5. Pour about 1 cup of flour onto the surface on which you will knead the dough. Spread the flour around a little. Turn the dough out onto the flour. Knead for 15-20 turns, adding flour as necessary, dough is somewhat elastic, but still a little sticky. Use this extra flour to scrape the sticky dough off your hands, too. When you are finished kneading, you should have a ball that is stiff, but elastic, and just slightly sticky to the touch. It will not be as elastic as yeast bread, and will be much heavier.

6. Divide the ball into two parts and pat into round shapes. Place on floured baking sheet, or in two well-oiled and floured loaf pans. If placed in loaf pans, gently flatten the tops with the palms of your hands. Brush tops with beaten egg for a shiny crust or brush with a thin layer of safflower oil for a softer crust.

7. Bake immediately at 350F for about 50 minutes, until knife or toothpick stuck in center comes out dry. Remove from pans and let cool. Keep the bread in the refrigerator and, if possible, heat each slice before serving. The bread tastes best warm, with fresh butter and honey.

Delicious and Nutritious Whole Wheat Bread-With Milk

Cholesterol Free
Egg Free
Suitable through Stage II

This variation of ***Delicious and Nutritious Whole Wheat Bread*** is made with milk for a slightly softer consistency.

expeller pressed safflower oil for greasing pans

extra whole wheat flour for flouring pans

1-1/2 c. old fashioned rolled oats

2 c. nonfat milk

1/3 c. unprocessed clover honey

1/3 c. expeller pressed safflower oil

3 c. whole wheat flour to start

3 tsp. baking powder

1/4 tsp. baking soda

1 tsp. sea salt

1-7 c. additional whole wheat flour

1 egg, beaten (optional)

additional expeller-pressed safflower oil for crust

1. Preheat the oven to 350F.

2. If using loaf pans, oil them well and flour them. If using cookie sheets, flour them. Set aside.

3. In a very large bowl, mix the oats, milk, honey and safflower oil. Let this mixture sit for a few minutes. While the wet mixture is sitting, combine dry ingredients in another bowl (3 c. flour, baking powder, baking soda, and salt). Mix thoroughly.

When oats are soft, add dry ingredients to wet. Stir well with a wooden spoon.

4. Add one cup of additional flour at a time, enough to make the dough manageable for mixing.   You are ready to knead when the dough is very heavy, and pulls away from the sides of the bowl as you mix it.   The dough should be the consistency of thick clay, but a little sticky. Your hands will get very sticky kneading the dough, but just enjoy the experience!

5. Pour about 1 cup of flour onto the surface on which you will knead the dough. Spread the flour around a little. Turn the dough out onto the flour.   Knead for 15-20 turns, adding flour as necessary, dough is somewhat elastic, but still a little sticky.   Use this extra flour to scrape the sticky dough off your hands, too. When you are finished kneading, you should have a ball that is stiff, but elastic, and just slightly sticky to the touch. It will not be as elastic as yeast bread, and will be much heavier.

6. Divide the ball into two parts and pat into round shapes. Place on floured baking sheet, or in two well-oiled and floured loaf pans. If placed in loaf pans, gently flatten the tops with the palms of your hands.   Brush tops with beaten egg for a shiny crust or brush with a thin layer of safflower oil for a softer crust.

7.   Bake immediately at 350F for about 50 minutes, until knife or toothpick stuck in center comes out dry. Remove from pans and let cool.   Keep the bread in the refrigerator and, if possible, heat each slice before serving. The bread tastes best warm, with fresh butter and honey.

Crunchy and Nutritious Whole Wheat Non-Yeast Bread

> *Milk/Casein free (with butter)*
> *Egg Free*
> *Suitable through Stage II*

This crunchy and hearty variation of *Delicious and Nutritious Whole Wheat Bead* makes a great tea bread, good enough for dessert, served with honey or fruit.

　　　expeller pressed safflower oil for greasing pans

　　　extra whole wheat flour for flouring pans

　　　1-1/2 c. old fashioned rolled oats

　　　2-1/2 c. water

　　　1/4 c. expeller pressed safflower oil

　　　1/4 c. melted butter (not margarine)

　　　1/2 c. unprocessed clover honey

　　　1/2 c. "Wheatena" or other whole wheat cereal

　　　3 c. whole wheat flour to start

　　　3 tsp. baking powder

　　　1/4 tsp. baking soda

　　　1 tsp. sea salt

　　　1-7 c. additional whole wheat flour

　　　1 egg, beaten (optional)

　　　additional expeller-pressed safflower oil for crust

1. Preheat the oven to 350F.

2. If using loaf pans, oil them well and flour them. If using cookie sheets, flour them. Set aside.

3. In a very large bowl, mix the oats, Wheateana, water, safflower

oil, melted butter and honey. Let this mixture sit for a few minutes. While the wet mixture is sitting, combine dry ingredients in another bowl (3 c. flour, baking powder, baking soda, and salt). Mix thoroughly. When oats are soft, add dry ingredients. Stir well with a wooden spoon.

4. Add one cup of flour at a time, enough to make the dough manageable for mixing. You are ready to knead when the dough is very heavy, and pulls away from the sides of the bowl as you mix it. The dough should be the consistency of thick clay, but a little sticky. Your hands will get very sticky kneading the dough, but just enjoy the experience!

5. Pour about 1 cup of flour onto the surface on which you will knead the dough. Spread the flour around a little. Turn the dough out onto the flour. Knead for 15-20 turns, adding flour as necessary, until the dough is somewhat elastic, but still a little sticky. Use this extra flour to scrape the sticky dough off your hands, too. When you are finished kneading, you should have a ball that is stiff, but elastic, and just slightly sticky to the touch. It will not be as elastic as yeast bread, and will be much heavier.

6. Divide the ball into two parts and pat into round shapes. Place on floured baking sheet, or in two well-oiled and floured loaf pans. If placed in loaf pans, gently flatten the tops with the palms of your hands. Brush tops with beaten egg for a shiny crust or brush with a thin layer of safflower oil for a softer crust.

7. Bake immediately at 350F for about 50 minutes, until knife or toothpick stuck in center comes out dry. Remove from pans and let cool. Keep the bread in the refrigerator and, if possible, heat each slice before serving. The bread tastes best warm, with fresh butter and honey.

Challah

Milk/Casein free
Suitable through Stage II

Challah is the traditional Jewish egg bread eaten on the Sabbath and holidays. Challah usually is braided, but on special holidays, the bread is shaped into a crown instead.

1-1/2 c. old fashioned rolled oats

2-1/2 c. water

1/2 c. expeller pressed safflower oil

1/2 c. unprocessed clover honey

2 large or 3 medium sized eggs

4 c. whole wheat flour or whole wheat pastry flour to start

4 tsp. baking powder

1/4 tsp. baking soda

1 tsp. sea salt

1-4 c. additional whole wheat flour or whole wheat pastry flour

1 egg, beaten (optional)

additional expeller-pressed safflower oil for crust

1. Preheat the oven to 350F.

2. Lightly dust a cookie sheet with flour. Set aside.

3. In a very large bowl, combine the oats, water, safflower oil, eggs and honey. Let the mixture sit for a few minutes to allow the oats to soften. While the mixture is sitting, combine dry ingredients in another small bowl (4 c. flour, baking powder, soda and salt). Mix thoroughly. When oats are soft, add the dry ingredients to the wet ingredients. Stir well with a wooden spoon.

4. Add additional whole wheat flour one cup at a time, mixing well after each addition, until the dough is the consistency of heavy wet clay. The dough should pull away from the sides of the bowl as you mix it. Now you are ready to knead.

5. Pour one cup of flour on the surface on which you will knead the bread. Turn out the dough. Knead for a few minutes until dough is somewhat elastic, but still a little sticky. If required, add extra flour to the challah. Knead for about 15-20 turns.

6. To shape the challah, make braids or a crown. To braid the challah: divide into six fairly equal parts. Knead each part separately; let them sit for a few minutes. Roll each part into a long rope, about 1 to 2 inches in diameter. Take three ropes. Lay them alongside each other. Press the tops together. Gently braid to the end of the ropes, then join ends. Press both ends under the loaves. For a crown shaped challah: divide the dough into two equal parts. Roll each part into a long, thick rope. Coil each rope of dough around itself until it looks like a crown, with a knot on top. Tuck the end under the loaf.

7. Place the loaves on the floured cookie sheet. If desired, brush tops with beaten egg for shiny crust. For a softer crust, brush with a thin layer of safflower oil. Bake immediately at 350F. for 30-60 minutes, until knife or toothpick stuck in center comes out dry. Remove from cookie sheet and cool.

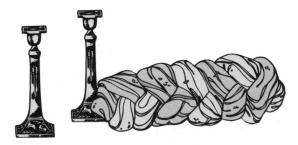

Pizza Bread

Milk/Casein free (with butter)
Egg Free
Suitable through Stage II

Crave pizza? This is the bread for you! The spices give the bread the sweetest hint of pizza flavor, but are mild enough to eat with other foods. If you want robust flavor, use one and one half to two times the amounts of basil and oregano. For an extra special meal, serve with *Thick 'N Chunky Tomato Soup.*

1-3/4 c. fresh tomato juice or pureed tomato

3-1/4 c. water

4 T. butter, melted

2 cloves garlic, chopped

3/4 c. expeller-pressed safflower oil

1/2 c. unprocessed clover honey

8 c. whole wheat flour + flour for kneading

2 T. baking powder

2 tsp. dried basil

2 tsp. dried oregano

2 tsp. sea salt

1/2 tsp. baking soda

1 egg, beaten and mixed with water for egg wash (optional)

*Preheat oven t*o 350F. *Flour* 2 cookie sheets. *Saute* the garlic in the melted butter and set aside. In a large bread-making bowl, *mix* the tomato juice, water and sauteed garlic together.   Add the oil and honey; mix well. *In a separate bowl, mix* the dry ingredients (flour, baking powder, herbs, salt and baking soda). Gradually add the dry mixture to the wet mixture. The dough will be sticky and very gloppy. *Turn the mixture* onto a well-floured board or counter. Separate into four pieces. *Knead* each piece about 10-15 times, working enough flour into the dough that it is workable and not too sticky, but not dry. *Shape* into round loaves. For a shiny crust, brush with egg wash. *Bake* at 350F for about 50 minutes, or until a knife or toothpick stuck into center comes out dry.

Crunchy Granola

Cholesterol Free
Milk/Casein Free
Egg Free
Suitable through Stage II

Great for breakfast and snacks. This freezes well.

5-1/2 c. rolled oats, or combination of grain flakes, such as oats, wheat, barley except rye

2 c. raw wheat germ

3/4 c. expeller-pressed safflower oil

3/4 c. clover honey (unprocessed)

Preheat the oven to 325F. *Mix* all ingredients well in a large bowl. Put in a 9x13 inch pyrex baking dish. *Bake* for about 35 minutes, turning the mixture every 10 minutes while baking. After removing the granola from the oven, be sure to turn it and scrape it loose while it is cooling, or you will get a cement-like mixture at the bottom of the baking dish. Line a bowl with wax paper and pour the warm granola into that bowl! Eat when it's cool.

Light 'n Flaky Whole Wheat Biscuits

Egg Free
Suitable through Stage II

1/2 c. butter at room temperature

2 c. whole wheat pastry flour to start

1 T. baking powder

1 tsp. sea salt

4 T. nonfat, non-instant milk powder plus 1 c. water

~ or 1 c. nonfat milk

additional whole wheat pastry flour for kneading

Preheat oven to 350F. *Mix* the flour, baking powder and sea salt together. If using non-fat, non-instant milk powder, mix it into the flour mixture. *Cut* the butter into the flour with a pastry blender or knives, until the size of sand grains. *Add* the milk, or, if using non-fat, non-instant milk powder, add the water. *Mix* well. Turn the dough out onto a floured surface. *Knead* with additional whole wheat flour for about 2 minutes, kneading in flour as necessary to make the dough very springy. Roll out to 1/2 inch thickness. *Cut* with a biscuit cutter or a drinking glass dipped in flour for round shapes or with cookie cutters dipped in flour for fun shapes. Place on a non-stick cookie sheet or on a lightly greased regular cookie sheet. *Bake* at 350F for about 12 minutes, or until the biscuits rise and start to brown. Makes about 2 dozen biscuits, depending on the size of the biscuits.

Whole Wheat Biscuits without Milk

Milk/Casein Free (with butter)
Egg Free
Suitable through Stage II

These biscuits are heartier than **Light 'N Flaky Whole Wheat Biscuits**, but still taste great.

1/2 c. butter

2 c. whole wheat pastry flour

1 T. baking powder

1 tsp. sea salt

additional whole wheat pastry flour for kneading

1 c. water

Preheat the oven to 350F. *Mix* the flour, baking powder and salt. *Cut* the butter into the flour mixture with a pastry blender or knives, until the mixture and butter resembles large grains of sand. *Add* the water. *Mix* well. *Knead* with extra whole wheat flour for about 2 minutes, until the dough is very springy. *Roll* out to 1/2 inch thickness. Cut with a water glass or biscuit cutter dipped in flour for round shapes or with cookie cutters dipped in flour for fun shapes. Place on a non-stick cookie sheet. *Bake* at 350F for about 12 minutes, or until the biscuits rise and start to brown. Makes about 2 dozen biscuits, depending on the size of the biscuits.

Light and Fluffy Pancakes and Variations

Milk/Casein Free (Non-Dairy Pancakes Variation 5) Suitable through Stage II

This recipe is an all time favorite of everyone who has tried it. We usually think of Sunday morning as the time for these simple and sweet cakes, but they make an excellent supper, too. They are so sweet that you won't even need syrup to top them off. I like to double or triple the recipe and freeze the pancakes, then reheat a few at a time for snacks.

1 c. whole wheat pastry flour

1 T. baking powder

1 c. nonfat milk

~ *or* ~ 4 T. non-instant, non-fat dry milk plus up to 1 c. water

1 egg

3 T. expeller-pressed safflower oil

2 T. unprocessed clover honey

Mix the flour, baking powder, and non-fat, non-instant milk (if using that). Make a well in the center. *Put* the egg, oil and honey in the well. If using regular milk, add the milk. If using milk powder, add 1/2 c. of water. Mix together. If the batter is too thick, add additional water a little at a time to the consistency you prefer. *Heat* an electric skillet to 325F, or heat a frying pan until a drop of water dances across the surface. When the pan is ready, *spoon* small amounts of batter on the ungreased skillet to form pancakes about 3 inches in diameter. *Cook* until golden brown on one side, then flip. To freeze: first cool the pancakes, then place in freezer containers. Enjoy!

Variation 1: Berry Cakes

Add 2 c. fresh blueberries or raspberries to the batter before cooking the pancakes

Variation 2: Apple Cakes

Add 2 c. fresh, finely chopped peeled apples to the batter before cooking

Variation 3: Spelt Cakes

Substitute Spelt Flour for Whole Wheat Flour, for less gluten and greater flavor

Variation 4: Stone Ground Whole Wheat Pancakes

Substitute stone ground whole wheat flour for whole wheat pastry flour. The pancakes will be grainier and have fuller flavor, but will still be light and fluffy.

Variation 5: Non Dairy Pancakes

Leave out the milk. Use 1/2 c. water instead. The pancakes will taste just as great, but will be less fluffy.

Honey Bran Muffins

Milk/Casein free
Suitable through Stage II

These all-purpose muffins are good to serve any time.

1 c. bran

1-1/2 c. water

1 egg

1/2 c. unprocessed clover honey

1/3 c. expeller-pressed safflower oil

1-1/2 c. whole wheat flour

2 tsp. baking powder

1/2 tsp. cinnamon (optional)

1/2 tsp. baking soda

1/2 tsp. sea salt

Preheat the oven to 400F. *Mix* the bran, water, egg, honey and oil in a small bowl. Let rest at least 5 minutes, until bran is soft. Meanwhile, *mix* the dry ingredients together in a large bowl. *Add* wet to dry ingredients, mixing as little as possible. *Pour* into muffin tins. *Bake* at 400F until a toothpick comes out dry, about 20 minutes. Makes about 18 regular sized muffins.

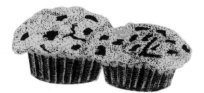

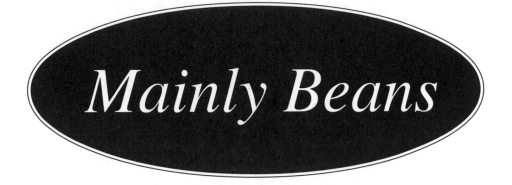

Mainly Beans

Beans are a staple of the combined yeast free, Wheat/Gluten Free, Milk/Casein Free diet. As you progress through the stages of the diet, you will incorporate more beans into your family meals. This chapter tells you how to cook great tasting beans. Be sure to look other places in this cookbook for additional recipes using beans! Here, we

~ explain how to purchase and cook beans

~ provide many excellent, easy bean recipes

The Basics of Beans

Beans are a staple of a yeast-free diet. Beans are high in fiber and nutrients, including calcium, and low in fat. They contain no cholesterol, gluten, yeast, or other offending substances.

Different beans have very different flavors and textures. When cooked, black "turtle" beans are firm and smooth; kidney beans are mild and soft; navy beans are very mild and almost sweet. There are several varieties of beans in addition to those just mentioned, including small red beans, garbanzo beans (chick peas), limas, Great Northerns, black-eyed peas, split peas and lentils, as well as even more exotic beans that you may find at health food and specialty stores.

Menu planning can be as simple as deciding what type of bean you will serve the next day (we call it "the *bean du jour"),* putting some of those beans in a slow cooker the night before, then draining, rinsing and cooking them according to an accept-able recipe before dinner. Beans even make great snacks—take a few from the slow cooker, rinse (if desired), and put on a little salt, oil, and tomatoes.

Many people avoid beans because of digestive gas. When cooked for a long time, as we recommend, the gas decreases. In addition, you will find that as beans become a steady part of your diet, you will experience much less gas. The slow cooking method described below helps to maximize flavor and minimize gas.

Purchasing Beans

Whenever possible, buy dried beans instead of canned beans, remembering the simple rule: if you don't prepare the food, you won't know what's in it. Moldy beans are quite common. Canned beans potentially contain beans that were moldy when canned, which spreads the mold to the entire can. Dried beans can be inspected to eliminate the especially bad ones.

Beans are best purchased in bulk from cooperatives or health food stores or grocery stores with high product turnover. If necessary, you can purchase prepackaged beans from supermarkets, but try to check on how fast these items turn over in the store.

Cooking Beans

For a family of four, measure out about 2-1/2 to 3 cups of whatever type of bean you are using. Look through the beans for discoloration. Discard beans that look noticeably different from the others in color, shape or texture, or have dark (moldy) areas. Also remove any dirt or stones. Rinse the beans.

We advocate two basic methods of cooking beans to use in dishes that are mainly beans, such as the ones in this chapter. You will find other delicious recipes for using beans in soups, sauces and other foods elsewhere in this cookbook.

The slow-cooker method and the quick soak method are the two best methods for cooking beans. We do not use the conventional slow overnight soak method because it increases the chance of fermentation. The slow-cooker method has advantages because it takes the least preparation time and involves the fewest boil overs. Slow cooking also decreases gas from beans.

Slow Cooker

This method works for the harder beans, such as kidney, black, small red, and garbanzos. Do not use it for navy beans or lentils—they will fall apart and you will have mush. Place the beans in the cooking part of a slow cooker. Cover the beans with about 3-4 times as much water as beans. Cover. Cook on high heat until the beans are soft, usually several hours or overnight. Reduce to low heat and continue cooking until you need the beans. If necessary, the beans can be cooked for as long as 48 hours, but we do not recommend cooking them for more than 24 hours. You may need to replenish the water every once in awhile. Drain the beans in a colander and rinse before using.

Quick Soak

The second choice method for cooking beans is the quick soak. Place 2-3 cups of beans in a large pot. Cover with sufficient water, according to the chart below. Bring to a boil. Remove beans from heat. Allow them to soak for an hour. Cast off the water and replace with fresh water, according to the chart below. Bring to a boil and cook for the amount of time shown in the chart below.

Beans (1 c. dry)	Amt. Water (in cups)	Cooking Time	Yield (cups)
Anazasi	3	2.5 hr.	2
Black Turtle	3	1.5 hr.	2
Garbanzo	4	4 hr.	3
Kidney	3	2 hr.	2
Lentils	2.5	45 min.	2
Navy	3	1.5 hr.	2

Using the Precooked Beans

Now that you have some cooked beans, what do you do with them? The recipes in this section are for main dishes that use beans. Other parts of this book also use beans, so be sure to visit those sections as well.

Our favorite easy way to serve beans is to stir-fry them or to serve **Hot Beans** as a snack. The stir-fry combinations are almost infinite.

You can also make leftover beans into burgers; you can use them in salads and soups. This recipe book should be considered a start, not an end-point, for your creativity. Here are some of our favorite recipes.

Hot Beans

Cholesterol Free
Gluten Free
Casein Free
Egg Free
Suitable through Stage IV

This very simple way to make beans takes about a minute to prepare and makes a great easy snack.

> Any amount of beans cooked according to directions in this book
>
> expeller pressed safflower oil
>
> sea salt
>
> Chopped fresh tomatoes (optional)

Place some beans on a plate. Pour over some safflower oil.

Sprinkle with sea salt, to taste. Add the fresh tomatoes, if desired.

Mix and eat.

Lemon Garbanzo Beans

Cholesterol Free
Wheat/Gluten Free
Milk/Casein Free
Egg Free
Suitable through Stage IV

This is one of the simplest recipes, yet so delicious you can serve it any time. Serves 3-4. Increase the recipe proportionally.

> 3 c. cooked garbanzo beans
>
> Juice of two fresh lemons
>
> Sea salt to taste
>
> 1 T. expeller pressed safflower oil

Mix all ingredients together. Taste; adjust lemon juice and salt.

Serve hot or cold.

Brazilian Black Beans

> *Cholesterol Free*
> *Wheat/Gluten Free*
> *Milk/Casein Free*
> *Egg Free*
> *Suitable through Stage IV*

This is an excellent dish to serve with **Spanish Rice** or **Rice with Tomatoes**. Accompany the beans with chopped fresh lettuce. Through Stage III, also chop up some oranges to accompany this dish.

2 "spring" onions (a white bulb onion with greens attached), *or* 1 bunch scallions with greens *or* 1 leek

2-3 cloves garlic

1 large tomato

2-1/2 c. dry black "turtle" beans, prepared according to directions in this book

expeller pressed safflower oil for frying

sea salt

Chop the onions and set aside. Chop the garlic and set aside. Chop the tomato and set aside. Drain the beans in a colander; rinse. *Heat* a "wok" or skillet very hot. Add enough safflower oil to cover the bottom of the wok 1/8 inch deep; use less for the skillet. When oil is hot, *add the onion*s; stir-fry them very quickly, about 1 minute. Then *add the garlic* and stir-fry until the garlic is golden brown, about 15 seconds. *Add the tomatoes* and continue stir-frying. *Mash* the tomatoes a little as you are cooking. When the tomatoes, onions, garlic and oil form a sauce, add about 1 cup of black beans. Mash the beans and stir. Cook about a minute longer. *Add* the rest of the beans and cook through without mashing. Add salt to taste. If beans begin to dry out, add 1/4 c. water. Boil off any excess water. Serve hot.

Garlic Beans

Cholesterol Free
Wheat/Gluten Free
Milk/Casein Free
Egg Free
Suitable for Stage IV

These beans are for garlic lovers only!

2-1/2 c. dry beans, prepared according to directions in this book

4 cloves fresh garlic

expeller pressed safflower oil for frying

sea salt

Drain the beans in a colander. Rinse. *Chop* the garlic and set aside. Heat a wok or skillet on medium heat for a few minutes. Add enough safflower oil to cover bottom of wok 1/8 inch deep; use less for skillet. *Heat* the oil until it is hot enough to cook the garlic without burning it. Add the garlic; stir-fry until it is golden brown, about 30 seconds. Add the beans and stir-fry. Add salt to taste. If the beans begin to dry out, add 1/4 cup of water. If you add too much water, boil it off. Remove from the wok or frying pan and serve. This recipe takes about 7 minutes from the time you drain the beans to the time you serve.

Five Minute Special Stir-Fried Beans

Cholesterol Free
Wheat/Gluten Free
Milk/Casein Free
Egg Free
Suitable through Stage IV

2-1/2 c. dry kidney, black, red or navy beans, prepared according to directions in this book

expeller pressed safflower oil, for stir-frying

sea salt to taste

1/4-1/2 c. water (optional)

Drain the beans in a colander. Rinse. Heat a wok or skillet on high heat. Add enough safflower oil to cover bottom of wok 1/8 inch deep. Use less for a skillet. When the oil is hot, *add* the drained beans. Keep turning the beans quickly so they do not burn. Add sea salt to taste. If the beans begin to dry out, add 1/4 cup of water. If you add too much water, boil it off. Remove from the wok or frying pan and serve. This recipe takes about 5 minutes from the time you drain the beans to the time you serve.

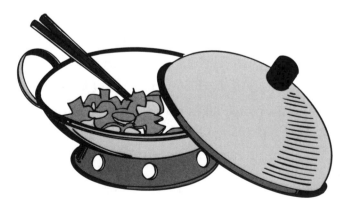

Savory Beans

Cholesterol Free
Wheat/Gluten Free
Milk/Casein Free
Egg Free
Suitable through Stage IV

2-1/2 c. dry beans, prepared according to directions in this book

2 "spring" onions (a white bulb onion with greens attached), *or* 1 bunch scallions with greens *or* 1 leek

expeller pressed safflower oil for frying

sea salt

Chop the onions and set aside. *Drain* the beans in a colander. Rinse. *Heat* a "wok" or skillet very hot. Add enough safflower oil to cover bottom of wok 1/8 inch deep; use less for skillet. Heat oil. When the oil is hot, add the onions; stir-fry very quickly, about 1 minute. *Add the beans* and cook through. Add salt to taste. If beans begin to dry out, add 1/4 cup of water. If you add too much water, boil it off. Remove from the wok or skillet and serve. This recipe takes about 7 minutes from the time you drain the beans to the time you serve.

Lentils, Plain and Simple

> *Cholesterol Free*
> *Wheat/Gluten Free*
> *Milk/Casein Free*
> *Egg Free*
> *Suitable through Stage IV*

Sometimes you just need "fast food," or something plain, simple and down home. Lentils hit the spot. They are quick and easy to make (taking only about 20 minutes to cook), plain and soothing to the palate.

   3 c. dried green or brown lentils

   1 T. sea salt, or more to taste

   7 c. water

Sort through the lentils, discarding obviously spoiled lentils. Rinse. Place the lentils in a pot with the salt and 7 cups of water. Cover. Bring to a boil; reduce to simmer; cook 20 minutes, or until lentils are soft. Adjust salt to taste. Remove from heat, or the lentils turn to mush. Serve immediately.

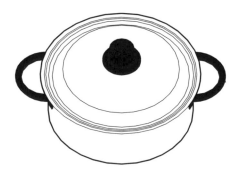

Beans Italiano

> *Cholesterol Free*
> *Wheat/Wheat/Gluten Free*
> *Dairy/Milk/Casein Free*
> *Egg Free*
> *Suitable for Stage IV*

Italian food lovers, welcome a new taste sensation. The herbs give the beans a fresh flavor, which nicely complements the onions and garlic. Takes about 10 minutes to make.

2-1/2 c. dry beans, prepared according to directions in this book

4 cloves fresh garlic

2 "spring" onions (white bulb onions with greens attached) *or* 1 bunch scallions, chopped (with greens) *or* 1 leek

expeller pressed safflower oil for frying

sea salt

1/2 tsp. dried basil *or* 2 tsp. fresh chopped basil

1/2 tsp. dried oregano *or* 2 tsp. fresh chopped oregano

Drain the beans in a colander. Rinse. *Chop* the garlic and set aside. Chop the onions and set aside. *Heat* a wok or skillet on medium heat. Add enough safflower oil to cover bottom of the wok 1/8 inch deep; use less for skillet. Heat the oil. When the oil is hot, add the onions; stir-fry for about 30 seconds. *Then add* the garlic and continue to stir-fry for about 30 seconds or until the garlic is golden-brown. *Add the herbs* and stir-fry about 15 seconds. Add the beans and stir-fry, mixing thoroughly. Add salt to taste. If beans begin to dry out, add 1/4 cup of water. If you add too much water, boil it off. Remove from the wok or frying pan and serve.

Tomato Beans

> *Cholesterol Free*
> *Wheat/Gluten Free*
> *Milk/Casein Free*
> *Egg Free*
> *Suitable through Stage IV*

Our favorite bean recipe, this one is deceptively simple. The tomatoes add moisture and sweetness to beans. Our guests consistently marvel at how great these refried beans are.

2-1/2 c. dry beans, prepared according to directions in this book

1 large tomato

expeller pressed safflower oil for frying

sea salt

water

Drain the beans in a colander; rinse. ***Chop*** the tomato and set aside. Heat a wok or skillet on high heat. Add enough safflower oil to cover bottom of the wok 1/8 inch deep; use less for a skillet. When the oil is hot, add the tomatoes. ***Stir-fry***. Add about 1/2 tsp. of sea salt. Continue stir-frying until the tomatoes have lost their shape and you have a sauce at the bottom of the wok. ***Add*** the beans and stir-fry to cook through. Add salt to taste. Mash the beans as they cook. If the beans begin to dry out, add a little water. If you add too much water, boil it off. Remove from the wok or frying pan and serve. This recipe takes about 10 minutes from start to finish.

Chinese Style Beans

Cholesterol Free
Wheat/Gluten Free
Milk/Casein Free
Egg Free
Suitable through Stage IV

2-1/2 c. dry beans, prepared according to directions in this book

4 cloves fresh garlic (optional)

2 "spring" onions (white bulb onions with greens attached) *or* 1 bunch scallions (with greens) (optional)

expeller pressed safflower oil for frying

sea salt

1 tsp. chopped fresh ginger

Drain the beans in a colander. Rinse. *If using* onions and/or garlic, *chop* and set aside. Heat a wok or skillet on medium heat. Add enough safflower oil to cover bottom of the wok 1/8 inch deep; use less for skillet. *Heat* the oil. When the oil is hot, *add* the onions or scallions and stir-fry until browned and soft. Then add the garlic and stir-fry for about 30 seconds or until the garlic is golden brown. *Add* the ginger and stir-fry for about 15 seconds more. Add the beans and stir-fry, mixing thoroughly. Add salt to taste. If beans begin to dry out, add 1/4 cup of water. If you add too much water, boil it off. Remove from the wok or frying pan and serve. This recipe takes about 10 minutes from the time you drain the beans to the time you serve.

Vegetarian Baked Beans

> *Cholesterol Free*
> *Wheat/Gluten Free*
> *Milk/Casein Free*
> *Egg Free*
> *Suitable through Stage IV*

This is a great recipe for plain ol' baked beans. These vegetarian beans are not baked, but simmered slowly—and are sooo delicious! Your children and guests will love them.

2 c. dry navy beans

water

3 very large or 6 medium tomatoes

2 tsp. sea salt

1/16 tsp. black pepper

1/2 tsp. dried oregano

3 T. freshly squeezed lemon juice

1 T. expeller pressed safflower oil

4 T. unprocessed clover honey

Put navy beans in a 3-quart pot and cover with water to within an inch of the top of the pot. Bring to a boil, then simmer. Cook the beans for about 1-1/2 hours until the beans have split open and are soft enough to eat, but are still firm. *Make the sauce* while the beans are cooking. Heat the oil in a skillet. Chop the tomatoes and add to the hot oil. Add herbs, salt and lemon juice. Bring to a boil, then simmer for at least 20 minutes. The sauce can simmer for several hours. The longer it cooks the better it tastes. *When the beans are done*, drain them and rinse in cold water. Add honey to the sauce. Mix well. Combine the sauce and the beans. Keep warm until ready to serve.

Lean and Tasty Bean Burgers

> *Cholesterol Free*
> *Wheat/Gluten Free*
> *Milk/Casein Free*
> *Egg Free*
> *Suitable through Stage IV*

This is another tasty favorite to make with leftovers, but requires some delicacy in handling the burgers. The recipe depends on your creativity and your stock of leftovers, so measurements are not exact. This recipe tastes great with *Super Bowl Salsa, Salsa Picante* or *Almost Barbeque Sauce*.

2 c. + leftover cooked beans *or* 1 c. dry beans, cooked according to the directions in this book

water as needed

1 tsp. mixed dried herbs (basil, oregano, dill and marjoram work well) per cup of cooked beans

sea salt to taste

expeller pressed safflower oil for frying

Preheat an electric skillet to 450F. If you do not have an electric skillet, preheat a heavy skillet, such as a cast iron skillet, until a drop of water dances across the surface. *Mash* the beans in a large bowl. A pastry blender or potato masher works well for this. Add water a little bit at a time, just enough to get a clay-like consistency. *Add the herbs*. Basil, oregano, dill and marjoram taste great either alone or in any combination. Add salt to taste. Pour enough oil into the skillet to cover the bottom to the depth of about a grain of rice. When the oil is hot, use a tablespoon to *scoop out* a little of the bean mixture, then *drop* it gently into the pan. *Gently press* down to form patties. Fry the burgers until they are crisp on one side, then gently turn them over and fry until crisp on the other side. Serve hot!

Lettuce Burritos

> *Cholesterol Free*
> *Wheat/Gluten Free*
> *Milk/Casein Free*
> *Egg Free*
> *Suitable through Stage IV*

For a fun, wheat-free and lower calorie alternative to traditional burritos, try this. You make it fresh at the table. Serve with *Tomato Rice* or *Spanish Rice* and *Salsa Picante* or *Super Bowl Salsa*.

   1 recipe *Refried Beans*, *Tomato Beans* or *Five Minute Special Stir Fried Beans*

   1 head romaine or iceberg lettuce

   2 c. chopped fresh tomatoes

   2 c. chopped fresh lettuce

Wash and separate the head of lettuce into leaves. If using romaine lettuce, break the spines of the larger leaves for easier rolling. Place some chopped lettuce, chopped tomatoes, and beans on a lettuce leaf. Roll and eat. Umm, Umm!!

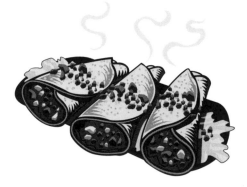

Frijoles Refritos

Cholesterol Free
Milk/Casein Free
Egg Free
Wheat/Gluten Free
Suitable through Stage III

These refried beans have a California-style Mexican flavor. They
go well with **Tomato Rice** or **Spanish Rice**, or served as **Whole
Wheat Burritos** or **Lettuce Burritos**.

> 3 c. dried pinto beans, cooked according to directions in this
> book
>
> 2-3 tsp. sea salt, plus more to taste
>
> 3 tsp. dried cumin powder
>
> 1/2 tsp. dried coriander
>
> expeller pressed safflower oil for frying
>
> water as needed

Drain and rinse the beans in a colander. Heat a large skillet or
wok until hot. Add enough oil to cover bottom lightly. When the
oil is hot, add beans, salt and spices. Mix well. Let the beans "re-
fry" for as much time as you have. Add water periodically to
keep the beans from drying out. If you add too much water, don't
worry. The water will just make a nice sauce.

Thick and Meaty Bean Burgers

Milk/Casein Free
Suitable through Level II

This is an all time favorite to make with leftovers. Although it uses no meat, the burgers are rich and tasty, giving you the feeling of eating beef. The measurements are not exact, but depend on your creativity, so relax and try different combinations of ingredients. This recipe tastes great served with **Super Bowl Salsa** or **Salsa Picante**. For an extra treat, serve with **French Fries Just like in the Restaurants**.

2+ c. leftover cooked beans, any type *or* 1 c. dry beans, prepared according to the method in this book

Any amount of leftover cooked grains, including oatmeal, rice, barley, bulgur, or whatever else you have

1-2 eggs

fresh raw wheat germ that has been kept in the freezer in both the store and your home

expeller pressed safflower oil for frying

1/2 tsp. mixed dried green herbs per cup of combined cooked beans and grains

sea salt to taste

Preheat an electric skillet to 450F. If you do not have an electric skillet, preheat a heavy skillet, such as a cast iron skillet, until a drop of water dances across the surface. **Mash** the beans in a large bowl. A pastry blender or potato masher works well. Add grains, if any. **Add a small** amount of wheat germ, about a tablespoonful. Add eggs one at a time, mixing after each addition until you have a consistency like thick clay. If the batter is too thin, add some more wheat germ until you can handle the batter. **Add seasonings**. Basil makes the burgers sweet. Basil plus oregano gives an Italian flavor. Dill makes them taste fresh and spring like. Add salt to taste. **Add enough safflower oil** to cover the bottom of the skillet generously. To **make the burgers**, either use the spoon-drop method (fill a tablespoon, drop the beans into pan, then flatten), or shape into burgers. If desired, **coat** the burgers with wheat germ for a crispier coating. When the oil is hot, place a pre-shaped burger or a spoonful of bean mixture into the oil. Cook only as many burgers at one time as your skillet can hold comfortably. Cook until crispy on one side; flip; cook until crispy on the other side. Place the cooked burgers on a heat resistant serving plate and keep warm until the rest of the burgers are cooked. Serve hot.

Garbanzo Zingers

Cholesterol Free
Wheat/Gluten Free
Milk/Casein Free
Egg Free
Suitable through Stage IV

This is a variation on **Lemon Garbanzo Beans**, for those who prefer a little zing in their food. Serves 3-4. Increase the recipe proportionally to serve more people.

3 scallions, chopped

2 cloves garlic, chopped

1 T. expeller pressed safflower oil

3 c. cooked garbanzo beans

Juice of two fresh lemons

Sea salt to taste

Heat the oil in a skillet. When hot, add the scallions and garlic. Saute until browned. Mix in the garbanzos and heat through. Add lemon juice and salt. Mix well; remove from heat and serve.Taste; adjust salt if necessary, and serve.

Jeweled Beans

> *Cholesterol Free*
> *Wheat/Gluten Free*
> *Milk/Casein Free*
> *Egg Free*
> *Suitable through Stage IV*

This dish looks and tastes delicious. The "jewels" are crunchy raw bell peppers. If you prefer softer, less vibrant jewels, you can stir-fry the vegetables before adding them. This dish is especially attractive using garbanzo beans.

1 large tomato

1 "spring" onion (a white bulb onion with greens attached), *or* 1/2 bunch scallions with greens *or* 1 leek

1 green or red pepper

2-1/2 c. dry beans, prepared according to directions in this book

expeller pressed safflower oil for frying

1/2 tsp. + more sea salt (to taste)

Chop the tomato and set aside. Chop the onion, scallions or leek and set aside. Chop the pepper and set aside. *Drain* the beans in a colander. Rinse and set the beans aside. *Heat* a wok or skillet on high heat. Add enough safflower oil to cover bottom of wok 1/8 inch; use less for skillet. Heat the oil. When the oil is hot, *add* the onions. Stir-fry them for a few seconds to about a minute and remove from the wok. Normally, the peppers will go into the beans raw and will be heated, but not cooked. If you prefer, stir-fry the peppers for about 1 minute. Remove. Add a little more oil to the wok, heat through, then *add the drained beans*. Stir-fry the beans, turning them quickly so all the beans get refried. Add 1/2 tsp. of sea salt to start; taste. Add more if you like. *Add the vegetables*. Cook through. If the beans begin to dry out, add 1/4 cup of water. If you add too much water, boil it off. Remove from the wok or frying pan and serve. This recipe takes about 10 minutes from the time you drain the beans to the time you serve.

Whole Wheat Burritos

Cholesterol Free
Milk/Casein Free
Egg Free
Suitable through Stage II

6 large whole wheat tortillas or chapatis

2 c. chopped fresh lettuce

2 c. chopped fresh tomatoes

1 recipe *Refried Beans, Five Minute Special Stir Fried Beans,* or *Tomato Beans*

Heat the tortillas or chapatis in a damp clean towel in the microwave. Place a large spoonful of beans in the center of a tortilla, then add lettuce and tomatoes. Fold up one side of the tortilla, then the two sides perpendicular, then fold the top down. Enjoy! Serve with *Super Bowl Salsa* or *Salsa Picante* and *Tomato Rice* or *Spanish Rice*.

Herbed Zucchini Lentils

Cholesterol Free
Wheat/Gluten Free
Milk/Casein Free
Egg Free
Suitable through Stage IV

This way of preparing lentils is quick and easy, taking only about 30 minutes, and tastes great.

3 c. dried green or brown lentils

2 bay leaves

1 T. sea salt, plus more to taste

3 medium zucchini, sliced

1 tsp. basil

7+ c. water

Sort through the lentils, discarding the obviously rotten ones, then rinse. Place all ingredients in a 3-quart pot. Cover; bring to a boil. Reduce to simmer and cook about 20 minutes, or until lentils are soft. Check the salt before serving. If desired, cook a little longer so the lentils begin to fall apart and get mushy. Serve hot!

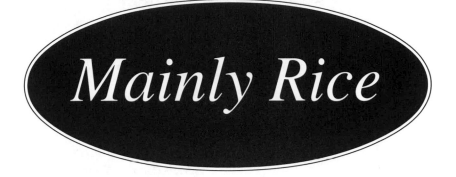

Mainly Rice

Rice is the staple food of most people in the world. It is the easiest food to tolerate, the least allergenic of the grains, and, as you will see, the best tasting! In this chapter, you will find recipes for tempting:

- *~ Fried Rice*
- *~ Rice with Spice*
- *~ Stuffing*

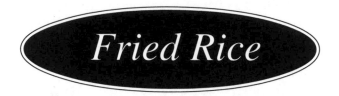

Vegetable Fried Rice

> *Cholesterol Free (without egg)*
> *Wheat/Gluten Free*
> *Milk/Casein Free*
> *Egg Free (without egg)*
> *Suitable through Stage IV*

Fried rice is versatile and can be as expressive as you are creative. We often use leftover rice to make different kinds of fried rice. This recipe is our basic vegetable fried rice, which you can vary according to what you have in your refrigerator and your imagination. Serves 6.

expeller pressed safflower oil for frying

2 c. chopped vegetables, using at least 2 different vegetables. Good combinations are: green beans, broccoli and red bell peppers; green beans, broccoli and carrots; zucchini, broccoli and green beans.

sea salt to taste

1 egg (optional)

2 c. cooked brown rice *or* 3/4 c. raw brown rice, cooked

Heat a wok very hot, or use an electric skillet set on the highest setting. *Add* 2 T. safflower oil. When oil is hot, but not smoky, *add* one of the vegetables; *stir-fry* quickly until done, about 30 seconds to 1 minute. *While stir-frying*, add a pinch of salt. *Remove* from the wok; set aside. *Add* more oil, if necessary.

Repeat individually with each of the remaining vegetables until you have used all of them. Then, if using egg, *scramble* the egg in a bowl. *Heat* 2 T. of oil in the wok. Put in a drop of scrambled egg. When the drop puffs up, pour in the rest of the egg, all at once. Lift the edges of the egg so the liquid part seeps under the solid part. When no more liquid is left in the center of the egg, turn it over. *Cook* until browned on the other side. *Remove* the pancake shaped egg and *cut* into small strips. If necessary, put a little more oil in the wok. *Add the rice*. Stir-fry a few minutes. *Add* 1/2 tsp. salt and continue turning. The rice should brown and become a little sticky. *Add* all of the cooked vegetables and egg. Stir; check salt. If the rice becomes too sticky, add a little water. Serve hot. Serves 6 hungry people.

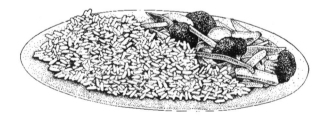

Chinese Style Fried Rice

Cholesterol Free (without egg)
Wheat/Gluten Free
Milk/Casein Free
Egg Free (without egg)
Suitable through Stage IV

This fried rice is similar to our Vegetable Fried Rice, but uses traditional Chinese seasonings of garlic and ginger to give it a lift. Serves 6.

expeller pressed safflower oil for frying

2 c. chopped vegetables, using at least 2 different vegetables. Good combinations are: green beans, broccoli and red bell peppers; green beans, broccoli and carrots; zucchini, broccoli and green beans.

sea salt to taste

1-2 cloves fresh garlic, minced

1/2 tsp. fresh, minced ginger

1/8 c. fresh minced leek

1 egg (optional)

2 c. cooked brown rice *or* 3/4 c. raw brown rice, cooked

Heat a wok very hot, or use an electric skillet set on the highest setting. **Add** 2 T. safflower oil. When oil is hot, but not smoky, **add one** of the vegetables; stir-fry quickly until done, about 30 seconds to 1 minute. **While stir-frying**, add a pinch of salt. **Remove** from the wok; set aside. **Add more oil**, if necessary. **Repeat** individually with each of the remaining vegetables you have. **Add** a small amount of oil to the wok. When hot, **stir-fry**

the garlic, ginger and leek until brown. Remove and set aside. *If using egg, scramble* the egg in a bowl. *Heat* 2 T. oil in the wok. Put in a drop of scrambled egg. When the drop puffs up, pour in the rest of the egg, all at once. Lift the edges of the egg so the liquid part seeps under the solid part. When no more liquid is left in the center of the egg, turn it over. Cook until browned on the other side. *Remove* the pancake shaped egg; cut into strips. Set aside. If necessary, *put a little more oil* in the wok. *Add* the cooked rice. Stir-fry a few seconds. Add 1/2 tsp. salt and continue turning. The rice should brown and become a little sticky. Add all of the vegetables and egg. Stir; check salt. If the rice becomes too sticky, add a little water. Serve hot.

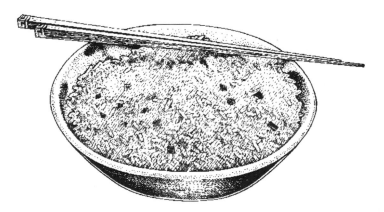

Zucchini Tomato Fried Rice

Cholesterol Free
Wheat/Gluten Free
Milk/Casein Free
Egg Free
Suitable through Stage IV

This dish is one of our favorites, a quick, easy and delicious way to use leftover rice. The tomatoes sweeten up the tart, fresh taste of zucchini.   Serves 6.

    4 medium zucchini

    2 tomatoes

    2 T. expeller pressed safflower oil

    1 tsp. sea salt, or sea salt to taste

    2 c. cooked brown rice

Slice the zucchini into thin slices. *Chop* the tomatoes into chunks, about one-half inch square. *Heat* a wok or frying pan on medium to high heat. *Add* two tablespoonsful of safflower oil. When oil is hot, add the sliced zucchini. *Stir-fry* until browned. *Add* the tomato. Cook through, until the tomato forms a sauce. Add the rice and heat through. Salt to taste.

Broccoli and Celery Fried Rice

Cholesterol Free
Wheat/Gluten Free
Milk/Casein Free
Egg Free
Suitable through Stage IV

This recipe takes two ordinary vegetables and turns them into one of the tastiest dishes you will find. Try it! Serves 6-8.

expeller pressed safflower oil for stir-frying

1-1/2 c. chopped broccoli

2 tsp. sea salt, or sea salt to taste

1 c. chopped celery

1 medium tomato, chopped

1 tsp. dried dill

1 tsp. dried basil

4-1/2 c. cooked brown rice

Heat a wok or frying pan on med-high heat. *Add* 2 tablespoons of safflower oil. *When oil is hot*, add the broccoli and a sprinkling of sea salt. Stir-fry until the broccoli is soft. *Add* the celery and stir-fry until celery is soft. *Add the tomato*, dill and basil. Cook through until the tomato forms a sauce. *Add* the rice and 1 tsp. of salt. Continue to stir-fry. *Add* oil if rice sticks to the wok. Test the seasonings; add salt if necessary.

Celery Dill Fried Rice

Cholesterol Free
Wheat/Gluten Free
Milk/Casein Free
Egg Free
Suitable through Stage IV

For the celery lovers, this fried rice tastes fresh and crunchy—a great way to use leftover rice. Serves 6.

   5 stalks celery

   2 T. expeller pressed safflower oil , plus more if needed

   2 c. cooked brown rice

   2 tsp. dried dill *or* 2 T. fresh dill, finely chopped

   1 tsp. sea salt

Chop the celery into small pieces, about 1/4 inch by 1/4 inch. *Heat* a wok or a frying pan very hot. *Add* 2 tablespoons of safflower oil. *Add* the celery. Stir-fry a few minutes until tender. *Add* the rice, dill and salt. Stir-fry until all ingredients are mixed through. Add small amounts of oil if the rice sticks to the pan. Serve hot.

Asparagus Fried Rice

> *Cholesterol Free*
> *Wheat/Gluten Free*
> *Milk/Casein Free*
> *Egg Free*
> *Suitable through Stage IV*

This is another variation on fried rice, especially great during asparagus season. It is simple yet tasty and delicious. Serves 6-8.

1 lb. asparagus

1 lg. clove garlic

2 T. expeller pressed safflower oil

3 c. cooked brown rice

1 tsp. dried basil

1 tsp. sea salt, or salt to taste

Cut off the tough ends of the asparagus, and chop into approximately one-inch lengths. Chop the garlic. Set asparagus and garlic aside. *Heat* a wok or a frying pan very hot. Pour in 2 tablespoons of safflower oil for stir-frying. *Add* the asparagus. Stir-fry a few minutes until tender. Add the rice, basil and salt. Stir-fry until all ingredients are mixed through. Test seasoning; add salt, if desired. Serve hot.

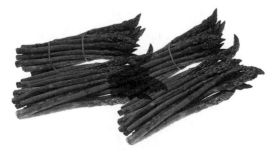

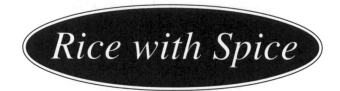

Rice-Ta-Touille

Cholesterol Free
Wheat/Gluten Free
Milk/Casein Free
Egg Free
Suitable through Stage IV

This very simple dish is a favorite of family and friends. It is a great dish to bring to potlucks. Serves 6-8.

    2 c. raw brown rice

    1 quart home-canned tomatoes, *or* 5 large tomatoes, peeled and chopped

    1-1/2 tsp. sea salt, or sea salt to taste

    2 medium zucchini, sliced

    1/8 tsp. black pepper (optional)

    4-5 c. water

Place all ingredients in a 3-quart saucepan. Cover and bring to a boil. Reduce heat; simmer covered for 50 minutes, or until rice is soft and fluffy. You might wish to check after about 20 minutes to make sure you have added enough water. When done, taste for salt. Add more if desired. Serve hot.

Spanish Rice

Cholesterol Free
Wheat/Gluten Free
Milk/Casein Free
Egg Free
Suitable through Stage IV

This is a favorite rice dish, great for guests. It goes well with just about everything. Serves 6.

2-4 T. expeller pressed safflower oil

1-1/2 c. raw brown rice

1 large or 2 medium fresh tomatoes, chopped

4 c. boiling water

1 tsp. sea salt

Heat oil in a 3-quart saucepan. The oil should be about as deep as a grain of rice. Put 2 to 3 grains of rice in the pot. *Heat* the raw rice until it toasts and is a nice brown color. *Add* remainder of rice all at once. You will toast this rice in the same manner.   Stir often; cook until rice begins to toast. *Add* the tomatoes and cook until the tomatoes start to get soft. *Carefully pour* in the boiling water. The water will steam and sizzle. Add the salt. Cover; bring to a boil, then reduce to simmer. Cook for about 50-60 minutes, without stirring. The rice will be soft when done. Serve hot.

Tomato Rice

Cholesterol Free
Wheat/Gluten Free
Milk/Casein Free
Egg Free
Suitable through Stage IV

This dish is a delicious, easy, no-fat-added version of **Spanish Rice**. Serves 6.

    1 large or 2 medium fresh tomatoes, chopped

    1-1/2 c. raw brown rice

    1 tsp. sea salt

    4 c. boiling water

Combine all ingredients in a 3-quart saucepan.   Cover. Bring to a boil, then reduce to simmer. Cook for about 50-60 minutes , without stirring. Serve hot.

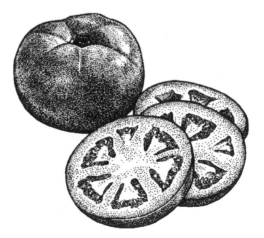

Savory Brown Rice

> *Cholesterol Free (using oil)*
> *Wheat/Gluten Free*
> *Milk/Casein Free*
> *Egg Free*
> *Suitable through Stage IV*

This is a favorite of family and friends. Serves 6.

2 leeks, chopped

3 T. butter or 3 T. expeller pressed safflower oil

2 medium zucchini, sliced

2 cloves garlic, chopped

4 T. chopped fresh parsley

1-1/2 c. raw brown rice

1 T. sea salt, or salt to taste

2 tsp. dried dill

4-1/2 c. water

In a 3-quart kettle, *saute* the leeks in the butter or oil until soft. *Add* the zucchini and garlic and cook until both are soft. Add the parsley. Add the rice. Add salt, dill and water. ***Bring to a boil***. Reduce heat and simmer for 50 minutes, or until rice is soft and fluffy.

Basic Brown Rice

> *Cholesterol Free*
> *Wheat/Gluten Free*
> *Milk/Casein Free*
> *Egg Free*
> *Suitable through Stage IV*

Brown rice goes with just about everything and forms the staple of a yeast free, Wheat/Gluten Free, Milk/Casein Free diet. One batch serves 6.

   1 c. raw long grain brown rice

   3 c. cold water (if pot does not seal well; 2 1/2 cups for tight sealing pots)

Put rice and cold water in a one-quart saucepan. *Cover*. Slowly bring the rice to a boil, over medium heat. When the rice begins to boil, lower to simmer. *Simmer*, covered, for about 50 minutes, or until water is absorbed. If your pot seals tightly, you can use 2-1/2 c. water. If your pot steams vigorously, you may need to use more water. Do not stir during cooking.

Celery Herb Rice

> *Cholesterol Free*
> *Wheat/Gluten Free*
> *Milk/Casein Free*
> *Egg Free*
> *Suitable through Stage IV*

This is a nice, subtly flavored herbed rice. It goes well with just about anything. Serves 4-6.

1-1/2 c. raw brown rice

3 stalks celery

1 tsp. dried marjoram

1 tsp. sea salt

5 c. water

Chop the celery. Place all ingredients in a 2-quart or larger saucepan. Cover and bring to a boil. Reduce to simmer. Cook 40-50 minutes, or until rice is tender.

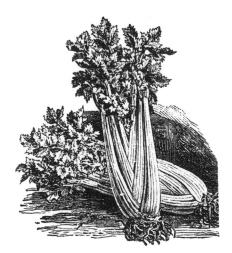

Herbed Brown Rice

> *Cholesterol Free*
> *Wheat/Gluten Free*
> *Casein Free*
> *Egg Free*
> *Suitable through Stage IV*

Making herbed brown rice instead of basic brown rice is a simple way to dress up an everyday meal. Serves 6.

2 c. raw brown rice

1 tsp. sea salt

1 tsp. dried basil

1/2 tsp. dill seed

1/2 tsp. dried rosemary

1/2 tsp. dried thyme

5-6 c. water

Combine the rice and seasonings. If using a rice steamer, ***add*** the amount of water you usually do for plain brown rice and cook according to directions for the steamer.   If cooking the rice on the stove top, add 5-6 cups of water. ***Cover***; bring to a boil; reduce to simmer. ***Cook*** for 50 minutes without stirring. Stir before eating.

Rice Burgers

Milk/Casein Free
Wheat/Gluten Free
Suitable through Stage IV

Looking for something to do with leftover rice? This is it! The recipe is designed to be multiplied. Ingredients are given for each 3/4 cup of cooked rice that you have. Each batch serves 2 hungry people.

> 3/4 c. cooked brown rice
>
> 1 large egg
>
> 1/4 tsp. sea salt
>
> expeller pressed safflower oil or butter for frying

Beat the egg with a fork. *Add* the rice and salt; mix well. *Heat* a skillet, add oil. When oil is hot, *drop* the rice/egg mixture into the oil by tablespoonsful. *Cook* each burger a few minutes on medium heat until the burger starts to brown. *Flip* over when the burger holds shape. Cook on the other side until lightly brown. Serve immediately. The number of burgers you make depends upon how large you make each one!

Sticky Rice

> *Cholesterol Free*
> *Wheat/Gluten Free*
> *Milk/Casein Free*
> *Egg Free*
> *Suitable through Stage IV*

This is extremely tasty rice with a nice, nutty flavor. This is a favorite among many of our guests. Serves 4-5.

1-1/2 c. raw short-grain brown rice

1/4 c. or less expeller pressed safflower oil

1 tsp. sea salt

3-4 c. water

Pour enough safflower oil in a 3-quart cooking pot to cover the bottom to the depth of a grain of rice. *Add* about 4 grains of rice. *Heat* on medium heat until the oil is very hot and the grains of rice start to brown. Avoid the temptation to turn the heat higher, or the oil will smoke and the rice will burn. When the grains of rice are brown, *add* the remaining rice all at once. Stir to coat the rice with oil. Let the rice *sizzle* in the oil, stirring frequently, until the rice starts to brown. This takes a minute or two. Be careful not to burn the rice. *Put on long oven mitts* to protect your arms, and carefully *add* the salt. *Add* 3-4 cups of water. If your pots are very tight, add 3 cups; if they leak steam, add 4 cups. **CAUTION: THE WATER WILL BOIL IMMEDIATELY. BEWARE OF STEAM.** *Cover* the pot; reduce heat to simmer. Cook about 50 minutes, until rice is cooked. Do not stir while cooking. Serve hot.

Fluffy Rice

Cholesterol Free (without butter)
Wheat/Gluten Free
Milk/Casein Free (without butter)
Egg Free
Suitable through Stage IV

This is an easy bake-ahead side dish, especially if you have an oven with an automatic shut off. The rice comes out very fluffy and does not burn. It takes at least an hour to bake, but can bake much longer. The longer the rice bakes, the fluffier it becomes, and it forms a nice crust around the edges. Serves 6.

2 c. raw brown rice

6 c. boiling water

1 tsp. sea salt

2 T. butter (optional)

Preheat oven to 350F. *Place* all ingredients into a pyrex or corning covered casserole dish, that will hold at least 2 quarts. The butter is optional, but makes the casserole taste even better. Stir. *Bake* for at least one hour, until rice is done. The rice bakes easily for two hours. If baking longer, be sure to check the water to make sure the rice is not sticking on the bottom. Add more water as necessary.

Baked Curried Rice

Cholesterol Free (without butter)
Wheat/Gluten Free
Milk/Casein Free (without butter)
Egg Free
Suitable through Stage II

This is a great dish to throw in the oven as you are baking other things for supper. It takes at least an hour to bake, but can bake much longer. The longer the rice bakes, the fluffier it becomes, and forms a nice crust around the edges. Very sensitive people may not be able to handle the curry powder. Serves 6.

2 c. raw brown rice

6 c. boiling water

1-2 tsp. sea salt

1 tsp. curry powder

2 T. butter (optional)

Preheat oven to 350F. *Place all ingredients* into a pyrex or corning covered casserole dish, that will hold at least 2 quarts. The butter is optional, but makes the casserole taste even better. Stir. *Bake* for at least one hour, until rice is done. The rice bakes easily for two hours. If baking for longer, be sure to check the water to make sure the rice is not sticking on the bottom. Add more water as necessary.

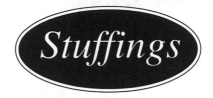

Marjoram Rice Stuffing

Cholesterol Free
Wheat/Gluten Free
Milk/Casein Free
Egg Free
Suitable through Stage IV

This is one of three delicious stuffings in this cookbook, very mildly seasoned, yet flavorful enough to grace any table. For a stronger flavor, use the greater amount of marjoram and the leek. This stuffing goes well with turkey, chicken, breast of veal, or just about anything else. Stuffs one medium sized turkey.

3 c. raw brown rice

6 stalks celery, chopped

1 large leek (optional), chopped

2-3 tsp. dried marjoram

2 tsp. sea salt or salt to taste

6 c. water + extra water if necessary

Place all ingredients in a 3-4 quart saucepan. Cover and bring to a boil. Reduce to simmer. *Cook* 40-50 minutes. Rice will be partially cooked. *Stuff* the body and neck cavities of the meat or poultry, close, and *cook* according to directions for that meat. Do not overstuff. The rice will expand during cooking. If you have extra stuffing, place in a casserole dish and add enough water to bring to the top of the rice. *Cover*. *Bake* in the oven with the turkey. Add juice from the meat or poultry to the casserole stuffing to get the full flavor. Serve hot!

Thanksgiving Stuffing

> *Wheat/Gluten Free*
> *Milk/Casein Free*
> *Egg Free*
> *Suitable through Stage IV*

All of the smells and tastes of Thanksgiving are rolled into stuffing. This rice stuffing satisfies anyone's palate for those traditional tastes. Precook the rice the night before you make the stuffing. Let it cool overnight in the refrigerator, so it will be easy to use when you make the stuffing in the morning. The rest of the stuffing takes about an hour to put together and stuff into the turkeys. This recipe makes a vat of stuffing, enough to stuff two medium sized turkeys, or one large and one small, and still have some left over. We prefer to have a lot of stuffing left over, even if only cooking a small turkey.

4 c. raw brown rice

8 c. water

4 T. expeller pressed safflower oil

2 large leeks

6 cloves garlic

5 c. chopped celery

2 tsp. dill seed

4 tsp. dried basil

1 T. dried marjoram

1 T. dried thyme leaves

2 tsp. celery seed

2 tsp. dill seed

1 tsp. ground sage

3 T. sea salt

Turkey drippings

1. Put the rice and the water in a large pot. Cover. Bring to a boil; reduce to a simmer. Cook for 50 minutes or until done. The rice will be slightly crunchy because it is only partially cooked. The rice will absorb juices from the turkey during cooking. Cool the rice to room temperature, then proceed with the rest of the recipe.

2. Heat the oil in a very large pot. Chop the leeks and garlic and add them to the hot oil. Saute for a few minutes, then add the celery. Saute until the celery is soft. Add all of the herbs and salt. Continue to saute. Add the rice and mix thoroughly. Cook through until you are ready to stuff the turkey(s).

3. Stuff the turkey(s) and roast according to your favorite roasting directions, usually 20 minutes per pound. We prefer coating the turkey skin with safflower oil, and roasting at 325F until done.

4. Put extra stuffing in an oven proof dish. Cover and refrigerate until there are enough turkey drippings to add to the stuffing. At that point, add at least one cup of liquid to the stuffing. More liquid will make the stuffing fluff up more. Bake covered at 325F for 30 minutes or more, to taste.

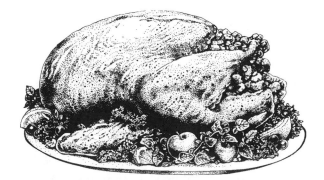

Basil Rice Stuffing

Wheat/Gluten Free
Milk/Casein Free
Egg Free
Suitable through Stage IV

This stuffing is great for Thanksgiving turkey or for other stuffed meats, such as breast of veal. It is especially good using fresh basil. Makes enough stuffing for one medium sized turkey.

3 c. raw brown rice

6 c. water

2-4 T. expeller pressed safflower oil for sauteing

2 cloves garlic, minced

1/2 to 3/4 c. chopped fresh basil leaves (packed) or 3 T. dried basil

giblets from turkey, chopped (optional)

1 tsp. sea salt or more, to taste

Cook the 3 c. rice in the 6 c. water by mixing in a 3-4 quart saucepan , bringing to a boil, and simmering for 50 minutes. *While the rice is cooking*, heat at least 2 T. oil in a very large frying pan. When hot, *add* the garlic and cook until browned but not burned. Add the basil and continue stirring. If desired, add the chopped giblets and cook through. Set aside until rice is done. Then, *add the rice* to the basil mixture. *Add* more oil if necessary to prevent sticking. Stir thoroughly. *Add the salt*. *Stuff* the body and neck cavities of the turkey, or other meat, close, and cook according to directions for those meats.   Do not overstuff. The rice will expand during cooking. If you have extra stuffing, place in a casserole dish and add enough water to bring to the top of the rice. Cover. *Bake* in the oven with the meat. Add juice from the meat to the casserole stuffing to get the full flavor. Serve hot!

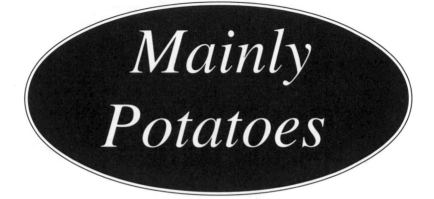

Mainly Potatoes

*Potatoes come in many sizes, shapes, colors and textures, and are among the most versatile of nature's foods. This chapter contains recipes whose main ingredient is potatoes, from lemon flavored baked potatoes to yams. Be sure not to miss the potatoes in our **Spectacular Soups** and **Super Salads**!*

Lemon Roasted Potatoes

> *Cholesterol Free*
> *Wheat/Gluten Free*
> *Milk/Casein Free*
> *Egg Free*
> *Suitable through Stage IV*

This dish is one of the all time most popular we have ever served. Although the dish is easy to put together, allow plenty of time to precook the potatoes. This is a good dish to start in the morning or even the night before to allow the potatoes to cool. I thank the Moosewood Restaurant for inspiring this recipe, in *New Recipes from the Moosewood Restaurant*.

8 medium sized "new" red potatoes

1 tsp. oregano

1-1/2 tsp. salt

1/2 c. freshly squeezed lemon juice

4 T. expeller pressed safflower oil

1 large or 2 small cloves garlic (optional)

Pre-bake the potatoes, whole and in the skins, either in the microwave or oven, until you can easily stick in a fork. *When the potatoes are cool* enough to handle, *preheat* the oven to 375F. Then *peel the potatoes* by slipping the skins off. *Take out* any bad spots, then *cut* them into about 1/2 inch cubes. *Place* in a 9x13 inch pyrex baking pan. *Pour* over the lemon juice, oil, salt and oregano. If using garlic, chop it finely and add to the mixture. *Mix well* until the potato cubes are covered with liquid. *Bake* at 375F for 50 minutes. *Stir* the mixture a few times during baking to make sure the potatoes roast evenly. When done, take out the pan and *let cool* for 30 minutes. Serve hot.

Dilled Potatoes

> *Cholesterol Free*
> *Wheat/Gluten Free*
> *Milk/Casein Free*
> *Egg Free*
> *Suitable through Stage IV*

You get a lot of mileage out of this surprisingly easy to make dish. The only difficulty is making enough to go around—it gets gobbled up too quickly! Ingredients are given per two potatoes. Make more or less, depending on the size of your family, appetite and skillet.

2 medium-sized white rose potatoes or red potatoes

2 tsp. butter

1/2 tsp. sea salt

1/4 tsp. dried dill weed

Pre-bake the potatoes in the oven or microwave, or use leftover boiled potatoes. Make sure they are cooked all the way through. Cool to a manageable temperature. *Peel* by slipping the skins off. *Slice* the potatoes in thirds lengthwise, then *slice* through the middle lengthwise. Then slice them crosswise into 1/8 inch slices. You will end up with small, thin pieces of potato. *Heat* a skillet, at least 9 inches in diameter, on medium-high heat. Melt the butter. *Add* the potatoes. *Mix* around. *Sprinkle* the salt over the potatoes; mix. *Sprinkle* the dill over the potatoes; *mix*. Let the potatoes *cook* a few more minutes, until they are a little brown and slightly crusty. Serve hot.

Light Potato Kugel

> *Cholesterol Free*
> *Wheat/Gluten Free*
> *Milk/Casein Free*
> *Egg Free*
> *Suitable through Stage IV*

Traditional potato kugel is delicious, and we miss it on an egg-free diet! This kugel is not as rich as the traditional kugel, but has a lot of flavor.

8 medium potatoes

4 T. expeller pressed safflower oil

1 tsp. sea salt

alternatives:

> 4 medium sized carrots or 2 medium zucchini
>
> *or* 1 bunch scallions, chopped, plus 1/4 c. chopped fresh parsley

Preheat oven to 375F. *Peel* the potatoes and place them in a bowl of cold water. *If using carrots or zucchini, peel* the carrots. *Grate* the carrots or zucchini on the "shredder" side of a four-sided hand grater. *Grate* 5 potatoes on the shredder side of the hand grater. *Grate* the other 3 potatoes on the next smaller grating side of the hand grater. You will get potato mush. *Mix* the potatoes and other vegetables together: either carrots or zucchini, or scallions plus parsley. *Add* the oil and salt; mix. *Oil* a 7x11 inch pyrex baking dish. *Pour* in the batter and smooth it down. Bake at 375F for 90 minutes, or until the kugel is golden brown on top. Serve warm or cold. The kugel's consistency will be slightly sticky, so use a serrated knife to cut the kugel into portions.

Traditional Potato Kugel

Milk/Casein Free
Suitable through Stage II

Potato kugel is a traditional Jewish dish that means potato
pudding. It is delicious on the Jewish holiday of Passover and all
year round. This dish is good hot or cold, so it's a good dish to
make in advance. It also freezes well after it's baked.

12 medium-sized red potatoes

2 carrots

1/3 c. whole wheat matzah meal or wheat germ (optional)

3 T. expeller pressed safflower oil

1 T. sea salt

5 scallions, chopped (optional)

2 - 4 large eggs

Preheat the oven to 350F. *Peel and grate* the potatoes. Make
sure your potatoes have no brown spots left. If any are green,
discard them. *Peel and grate* the carrots. In a large bowl, *mix* the
grated potatoes, carrots, matzah meal or wheat germ (optional),
oil, salt and scallions (optional). *Add* the eggs last, one at a time.
The batter should be easy to mix and wet, but not soupy. Adjust
the amount of eggs for this consistency. If you get a soupy
mixture, add a little more matzah meal or wheat germ. When all
ingredients are mixed, *place* in greased 7x11 or 9x13 inch pyrex
baking pan, whichever works better for you. *Bake* at 350F for at
least an hour, or until potatoes are cooked thoroughly.

French Fries Just Like in the Restaurants, but Better

Cholesterol Free
Wheat/Gluten Free
Milk/Casein Free
Egg Free
Suitable through Stage IV

Kids love french fries. Most restaurant french fries are unacceptable on a yeast free diet because the restaurants do not use acceptable fat for frying, and/or fry other foods in the same fat, contaminating it; and/or use fat for days at a time. These french fries work best with Idaho potatoes. Allow about an hour to cook. You can do other things while these are cooking, tending to the french fries from time to time. You can prepare the potatoes in advance, storing them completely covered in a bowl of cold water until ready to use.

> 6 large Idaho potatoes, or 1 large potato per person
>
> expeller pressed safflower oil for frying
>
> electric skillet or deep fryer
>
> sea salt

Peel the potatoes and clean them, *cutting* out any eyes, bruises or green spots. Place peeled potatoes in a bowl of cold water while preparing the rest. *Slice* the potato into strips about 1/4 -3/8 inch wide on all sides. *Cut* into the kind of lengths you like to eat. *Place* the sliced potatoes into cold water until ready to use. You can start to cook some potatoes while you are cutting the rest. These take a long time to cook. *Heat* oil in the electric skillet, about 1/2 inch deep, on a setting of 350F, or heat the recommended amount of oil in a small deep fryer. Use only fresh oil. *When the oil is hot, place* about a handful of potato pieces in the oil. ***Cooking*** more at one time does not save time in the long run, because each batch of potatoes will take longer to ***cook.*** ***Cook*** on one side until browned, then turn by using two forks, holding one in each hand. If you keep the oil at about 350F, the potatoes will not burn. When browned all over, ***remove*** from skillet with the forks or a slotted spatula or spoon. ***Place*** on a cooling rack placed over a brown paper bag, to drain. Do not ***drain*** directly on paper towels or paper bags, as that makes the french fries soggy. ***When drained, place*** on a plate. Salt. After you have ***removed*** one batch, place another batch in to cook. Keep the french fries warm in a 200F oven. ***Try*** to keep your snackers from eating all of them before the french fries get to the table!

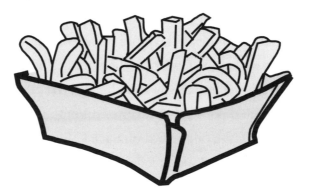

Quick & Easy French Fries

Cholesterol Free
Wheat/Gluten Free
Milk/Casein Free
Egg Free
Suitable through Stage IV

Craving french fries without the time for *French Fries Like in the Restaurants*? Try these. Increase the recipe as needed for your hungry appetites.

> 1 large Idaho potato or 2 medium sized red potatoes
>
> or a similar amount of other great tasting potatoes
>
> expeller pressed safflower oil for frying
>
> sea salt to taste

Peel the potatoes and *cut* out any brown spots or eyes. *Dice* into 1/2 inch cubes, or small strips. *Place* on a plate and *microwave* on high for about 4 minutes. The more microwaving you do, the less frying you need to do. *Covering* the potatoes before microwaving produces less crispy french fries. *Heat* a small skillet to medium and pour a thin layer of oil onto it. *Heat* the oil. Place the potatoes in the oil; brown on each side. When crisp and brown, *remove* from the skillet, place on plate, and salt to taste. *Serve* immediately.

Mashed Potatoes

> *Wheat/Gluten Free*
> *Milk/Casein Free*
> *Egg Free*
> *Suitable through Stage IV*

Everyone loves mashed potatoes, any time, any day.

> 6-8 large red potatoes
>
> water
>
> butter to taste
>
> sea salt to taste

Peel the potatoes, *cutting* out brown spots and eyes. *Cut* into small chunks. *Place* in a cooking pot. If the pot is of good quality, and you can be sure the water will not boil away, *fill* the pot about 1/4 full with water. If not, *cover* the potatoes with water. *Cover* the pot. Bring to a *boil* and reduce to a slow boil; *cook* until you can easily stick a fork into the potatoes. When potatoes are done, *place* a colander over a large bowl. *Pour* the potatoes and water into the colander. *Save* the cooking water. *Put* the potatoes in another bowl, or back in the pot. *Mash* them with a potato masher, *adding* as much cooking water as necessary to achieve a very smooth consistency. *Do not use* an electric mixer. The potatoes will get too pasty. Starting with about 1 T. of butter, *mix* in butter and salt to taste. Serve piping hot.

Hash Browns

> *Wheat/Gluten Free*
> *Milk/Casein Free*
> *Egg Free*
> *Suitable through Stage IV*

This recipe is one of our favorites. Our son usually eats 2-3 batches daily! This recipe can be made in less than 20 minutes and is great for feeding hungry children quickly.

>   2 medium Russet potatoes
>
>   1 T. butter
>
>   1 T. expeller pressed safflower oil
>
>   1/4 - 3/8 teaspoon salt, plus more to taste

Set a frying pan on the stove to begin heating at medium-low heat. While the frying pan is heating, *peel* the potatoes, making sure there are no dark spots anywhere. *Cut* the potatoes in half both lengthwise and across to make sure there are no bad spots. *Grate* the potatoes on the standard "shredder" side of a four sided grater. *Put* butter and safflower oil into the frying pan. After butter sizzles and melts *put* in grated potatoes. *Sprinkle* on the salt. *Turn* potatoes over after potatoes begin to brown. After first turning, *turn* potatoes about every two minutes to make sure all 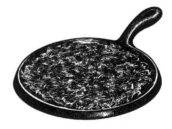 potatoes *cook evenly*. Potatoes are done when they are brown on both sides and cooked through. At a heat setting which browns but does not burn the potatoes, these potatoes take about 12 minutes to cook. *Test* for salt; *serve* piping hot!

Soft & Spicy Potato Latkes

Milk/Casein Free
Suitable through Stage II

This recipe is a variant on one we found in a children's book. The latkes are soft and spicy, and taste delicious.   Serve with **Pear Sauce** or **Cranberry Lemon Sauce, Cranberry Pear Sauce** or **Cranberry Fruit Sauce**.

5 red potatoes

6 scallions

3 T. whole wheat pastry flour

2 eggs

2 tsp. sea salt

1/4 tsp pepper

1 tsp. lemon juice

2 tsp. fresh chopped parsley

expeller pressed safflower oil for frying

Peel the potatoes, *cutting* out any brown spots and eyes. *Grate* the potatoes by hand or with a food processor. Then, *process* about 1/2 of the potatoes in a food processor or blender, *adding* the eggs. *Process* until smooth. *Add* scallions and process again. *Add* blended mixture to remaining grated potatoes, *mix* well, then *add* the rest of the ingredients. *Heat* electric skillet on highest setting. *Heat* some oil in skillet. *Drop* latkes by small spoonfuls onto skillet. When golden brown, *flip* over and brown on other side. *Serve* hot. If you are not serving directly from the frying pan, *drain* latkes on brown paper bags or paper towels. Keep the latkes warm in the oven at 200F.

Soft & Spicy Potato Latkes- Without Wheat or Eggs!

Cholesterol Free
Wheat/Gluten Free
Milk/Casein Free
Egg Free
Suitable through Stage IV

Most latkes are made with eggs and a little bit of flour, but these latkes are free of both. What holds them together? The natural potato starch that comes from processing some of the grated potatoes. These are delicious, light and airy. Your family and friends will love them. Serve with *Pear Sauce* or *Cranberry Lemon Sauce*.

5 potatoes (red or Idaho)

6 scallions

2 tsp. sea salt

1/4 tsp pepper

1 tsp. lemon juice

2 tsp. fresh chopped parsley

expeller pressed safflower oil for frying

Peel the potatoes, *cutting* out any brown spots and eyes. *Grate* the potatoes by hand or by food processor. Then, *process* about 1/2 of the potatoes in a food processor or a blender. Process until just slightly lumpy. *Add* scallions to the food processor and *process* again. *Add* blended mixture to remaining grated potatoes and add rest of ingredients. *Heat* electric skillet on highest setting. *Heat* some oil in skillet. *Drop* latkes by small spoonfuls onto skillet. When golden brown, *flip* over and brown on other side. *Serve* hot. If you are not serving directly from the frying pan, *drain* latkes on brown paper bags or paper towels. *Keep* the latkes warm in the oven at 200F.

Crispy Traditional Potato Latkes

Milk/Casein Free
Suitable through Stage II

A traditional Channukah dish, these potato pancakes are great year round. They are hot, crispy and delicious. Serve with *Pear Sauce* or *Cranberry Lemon Sauce*, *Cranberry Pear Sauce* or *Cranberry Fruit Sauce*.

8 large red potatoes

4 fresh eggs

1/4 c. matzah meal or whole wheat flour

2 tsp. sea salt

Lots of expeller pressed safflower oil for frying

Peel the potatoes and *cut* out any discolored spots. *Grate* the potatoes using a hand grater. I have found that a food processor grater does not shred the potatoes thin enough to get the best texture and flavor. *Beat* in the eggs, one at a time, to avoid too much liquid. *Add* the matzah meal or flour and the salt. The mixture should have the consistency of thick pancake batter. If it is too soupy, *add* matzah meal. If it is too thick, *add* an egg and more potatoes if necessary. *Adjust* salt.

The secret to crispy latkes is a hot skillet. *Heat* a skillet very hot, preferably an electric fry pan set at the highest setting, 450F. *Add* about 1/4 inch of oil. *Heat* the oil very hot. *Mix* the batter; drop in by tablespoonfuls. *Flatten* each latke so it cooks more evenly. *Cook* until crispy brown on one side, then *flip* over and cook the same on the other side. This takes time. *Adjust* the heat of the pan so the latkes do not *burn.*

Crispy Potato Latkes Without Eggs or Wheat

Cholesterol Free
Wheat/Gluten Free
Milk/Casein Free
Egg Free
Suitable through Stage IV

Channukah means potato pancakes (latkes). We were not about to give up latkes simply because we couldn't use the matzah meal and eggs required for traditional ones. What we devised were simply the lightest and most delicious latkes that can be made all year round. We have found that our guests prefer these latkes to traditional ones. One recipe makes enough latkes for 5 hungry people. Serve with *Pear Sauce* or *Cranberry Lemon Sauce*.

> 6 large russet (Idaho) potatoes
>
> safflower oil for frying
>
> salt to taste

Peel the potatoes and *cut* out any bad spots. *Grate* four of the potatoes on what we call the "regular" side of the grater (on a standard four-sided grater, this is the side most people use. It is smaller than the slicing side, but larger than any of the other sides). *Grate* the remaining two potatoes on the next smaller side. You might find that mashing the raw potato around in a circle against the edges is the most efficient way to do this. You will get mush. *Mix* all of the grated potatoes in a large bowl, including any liquid from the potatoes. *Add* salt to taste and mix. *Heat* an electric frying pan to 450F or a regular frying pan hot enough that a drop of water dances across the surface. *Add* oil to the depth of about a latke. When the oil is hot, *drop* large spoonfuls of the potato mixture into the oil and *flatten* each drop to form the pancakes. **Cook** until browned on one side, then *flip* and cook until browned on the other side. As each batch is done, **lift** from the frying pan and tap off excess oil. Place in a pyrex pan without blotting the oil. Latkes will get soggy if you blot. Keep the latkes warm at 175F-200F. Serve hot!

Microwave Baked Yams

Cholesterol Free
Wheat/Gluten Free
Milk/Casein Free
Egg Free
Suitable through Stage IV

Yams satisfy that desire to taste sweet things. They also fill you up, have no added fat (unless served with butter), are good complex carbohydrates and are relatively low in calories.

Any number of large, firm yams or sweet potatoes

Wash the yams thoroughly. **Prick** them with a fork. **Wrap** each yam tightly in plastic wrap that is microwave safe, or **place** all of the yams in an oven bag and seal it according to manufacturer directions. **Microwave** on high for approximately 5 minutes per yam, but **check** after 10 minutes even for a large number of yams. If they are soft and squeezable, they are done. If not, **microwave** 3 minutes at a time until the yams are soft. When you know how long your microwave takes to bake the yams, make a note so you can repeat this easily.

Personal note: My microwave takes _____ min. to bake _____ (number) of yams on high setting.

Baked Yams

> *Cholesterol Free*
> *Wheat/Gluten Free*
> *Milk/Casein Free*
> *Egg Free*
> *Suitable through Stage IV*

Some people prefer home baked yams to *Microwave Baked Yams*. They are just as easy, but take a little longer to bake.

Any number of large, firm yams or sweet potatoes
Canola oil no-stick cooking spray or safflower oil (optional)

Preheat oven to 375F. *Scrub* the potatoes. Either: *wrap* each potato in aluminum foil and place all directly in the oven, or lightly *grease* a cookie sheet with cooking spray or oil and *place* the plain potatoes on the cookie sheet, then in the oven. *Bake* for at least one to one and a half hours, until yams are soft to the squeeze. You may want to turn them over half way through cooking. *Serve* them as is, piping hot from the oven. *Cut* open and *scoop* out insides. *Top* with butter, if desired. Leftovers can be cut up into individual portions and frozen for later use.

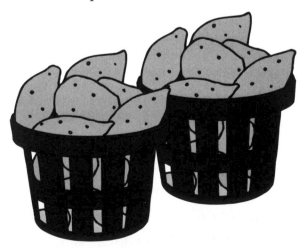

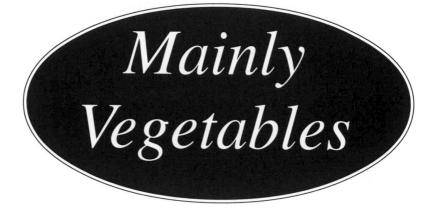

Mainly Vegetables

Vegetables can be exciting additions to your meal, whether as main dishes or side dishes. Almost all of our recipes use vegetables of one kind or another, but this chapter is devoted to recipes using vegetables as their main ingredient. In this chapter, you will find ideas for many types of vegetable dishes, from stir-fries to casseroles, from winter squash to tomato pie.

Braised Eggplant

Milk/Casein Free
Suitable through Stage II

1/4 c. plus 2 T. whole wheat pastry flour

2 large eggs

1/3 c. water, plus a few drops water

1/4 tsp. sea salt

1/4 tsp. pepper

1 large eggplant

expeller pressed safflower oil for cooking

Peel and slice the eggplant into 1/8 inch thick slices. If the eggplant is very large, cut each slice into halves or quarters. Set aside. *Make a batter* with the eggs, 1/3 c. water, salt, pepper and flour. *Heat* oil in a wok until hot enough that a drop of the batter cooks almost instantly. *Dip* the eggplant, one piece at a time, immediately prior to cooking that piece. *Cook* a few pieces at a time in the wok. When browned on one side, *turn* the eggplant over and cook the other side.   The eggplant is cooked when it is fork-tender.   *Remove* from the wok and *drain* by placing on a wire rack or in a colander standing over brown paper bags. This will keep the eggplant crispier than blotting it with paper towels. When all of the eggplant is cooked, serve piping hot.

Stir-Fried Eggplant with Garlic

> *Cholesterol Free*
> *Wheat/Gluten Free*
> *Milk/Casein Free*
> *Egg Free*
> *Suitable through Stage IV*

For eggplant lovers only, a lower fat, gluten, milk and egg free version of **Braised Eggplant .**

2 large eggplants, preferably Sicilian eggplant for milder flavor

2 large cloves garlic

sea salt to taste

expeller pressed safflower oil for stir frying

Preheat oven to 350F. **Cut** the eggplant into strips approximately 1/8 inch thick by 2 inches long by 1/2 inch wide. Set aside. **Lightly oil** two cookie sheets. Lay the eggplant strips in a single layer on the cookie sheets. Sprinkle lightly with salt. Cover loosely with aluminum foil. **Bake** at 350F for 30 minutes, or until the eggplant is soft. While the eggplant is baking, **mince** the garlic and set aside.   Remove the eggplant from the oven when done. **Heat** a small amount of oil in a wok or heavy frying pan. When the oil is hot, **add** the garlic and quickly stir-fry so the garlic browns, but does not burn. If the pan gets too hot, shove the garlic up a side of the wok and remove the wok from the heat to allow the oil to cool a minute or two. When the garlic is brown, **add** the eggplant and stir-fry for a few minutes. Add salt to taste. Serve hot.

Stir-Fried Zucchini with Tomatoes

Cholesterol Free
Wheat/Gluten Free
Milk/Casein Free
Egg Free
Suitable through Stage IV

2 medium zucchini

1 small tomato

3 T. expeller pressed safflower oil

1/2 tsp. sea salt, or salt to taste

Slice the zucchini as thinly as you can, the thinner the better. Set aside. **Chop** the tomato into small pieces. **Heat** the safflower oil in a wok or frying pan. When the oil is very hot, add the zucchini. **Stir fry** until browned and at least some are crisp. Add the tomatoes; continue to stir fry until the tomatoes are cooked through. Add salt to taste. Serve hot.

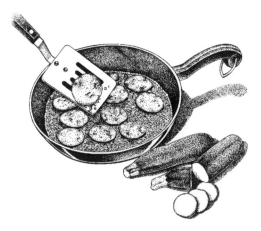

Spicy Flower

Cholesterol Free
Wheat/Gluten Free
Milk/Casein Free
Egg Free
Suitable through Stage IV

Spicy Flower makes the ordinary beautiful. Our daughter created this recipe for children to use.

1 medium tomato

1 zucchini, thinly sliced

expeller pressed safflower oil for sauteeing

1/2 c. cooked brown rice

large pinch of dried basil

large pinch of dried thyme

large pinch of dried oregano

Cut the tomato into thin, triangle shaped, bite-sized pieces. *Saute* the zucchini in safflower oil until it is browned. *Sprinkle* with basil. Remove from heat and cool. *Place* the cooked rice in the center of a dinner plate or round serving plate. Then, with a fork, *lay the zucchini* around the rice in a ring. Continue laying the zucchini until it is all gone. *Surround* the zucchini rings with the tomato pieces. *Sprinkle* thyme over the tomatoes, and oregano over the rice. This is as fun to eat as it is to serve.

Mini Tomato Pie

> *Cholesterol Free*
> *Wheat/Gluten Free*
> *Milk/Casein Free (with butter)*
> *Egg Free*
> *Suitable through Stage IV*

This pie is surprisingly sweet and delicious. Serve as a side dish or dessert.

1 large or two small tomatoes

1/4 c. potato flour

1/4 c. brown rice flour

1/2 stick butter (1/4 cup)

ice water

Preheat the oven to 350F. *Chop* the tomatoes into small pieces and set aside. In a large bowl, *combine* the flours. Crumble in the butter and blend the mixture with knives or a pastry blender until small pea-sized shapes form. Throw in ice-water, about a tablespoonful at a time, until you can shape this pastry into a pie crust. *Press* out the crust thinly into muffin tins. *Distribute* the chopped tomatoes among the muffin cups. *Crumble* some crust over the tomatoes. *Bake* at 350F for 30 minutes. Cool before serving.

Spaghetti Squash Italiano

> *Cholesterol Free*
> *Wheat/Gluten Free*
> *Milk/Casein Free*
> *Egg Free*
> *Suitable through Stage IV*

Spaghetti squash is a great alternative to pasta, low calorie and filling. This dish has a pizza-like taste, like making the spaghetti and sauce all in one. Start cooking at least 1-1/2 hours before you plan to serve.

1 large or 2 medium-sized spaghetti squash

3 medium zucchini

1 red bell pepper

3 cloves garlic

1-1/2 tsp. dried oregano

1-1/2 tsp. dried basil

sea salt to taste

expeller pressed safflower oil for sauteing

Cut the squash in half, preferably lengthwise. Scoop out seeds and clean out the obviously stringy pulp (the edible part of the squash is less stringy). *Cook the squash:* **Stovetop directions:** place open side down into 2" water, cover, and boil until inside is soft. **Oven Directions:** place open side down on a greased cookie sheet. Bake at 350F for about 45 minutes. **Microwave directions:** microwave whole squash on "high" in a small amount of water for 7-10 minutes. *Continue*: scoop out the fleshy part of the squash from the shell. This will resemble spaghetti. *Slice* the zucchini, chop the peppers and garlic. *Saute* the vegetables and garlic in a small amount of oil. *Mix* all ingredients with the spaghetti squash. Check seasonings, heat through (if necessary) and serve hot.

Basic Chinese Stir-Fried Vegetables

Cholesterol Free
Wheat/Gluten Free
Milk/Casein Free
Egg Free
Suitable through Stage IV

This recipe is a basic stir-fry, which you can vary by using different vegetables, or changing the amount of garlic and ginger you use. If you do not like ginger or garlic, leave them out! The dish will be even more delicious to you.

3 c. chopped or sliced mixed vegetables each chopped separately and put on a separate plate

1-2 cloves garlic

1/2 - 1 tsp. fresh, chopped ginger

1/3 c. chopped leek

expeller pressed safflower oil for frying

sea salt to taste

Choose your vegetables to create varied shapes and textures. Good choices include mixtures of green beans, broccoli, zucchini, yellow summer squash, red and/or green bell peppers, carrots (for those who like a sweet stir fry), or other vegetables. Do not use mushrooms or sprouts. Avoid snow peas and sugar snap peas unless you know for sure they are not mold contaminated. *Cut* green beans and broccoli into 1/2-inch pieces. Cut zucchini and yellow squash in half lengthwise, then into thin slices. Cut bell pepper and carrots into thin strips, about 2 inches long and 1/8 inch wide. *Make sure you place* each vegetable on a separate plate. *Chop* garlic, leek and ginger and mix together. *Heat* a wok until it is hot. Add about 2 T. of oil. Heat, but do not smoke it. ***Cook*** one vegetable at a time. Put the first vegetable in the wok, add a pinch of salt, then stir fry, mixing constantly. Cook about 30 seconds to a minute, a little longer for zucchini and yellow squash, then ***remove*** and place on a plate. Then ***cook the second vegetable***, and so on. You may need to add oil between vegetables. After cooking all the vegetables, you will cook the seasonings. If necessary, add a little more oil to the wok. Add the ginger, garlic and leek, stir frying quickly. Add back the rest of the cooked vegetables. Stir. Check the salt. If necessary, add salt 1/2 tsp. of salt at a time to taste. ***Serve*** piping hot alone or over ***Basic Brown Rice***.

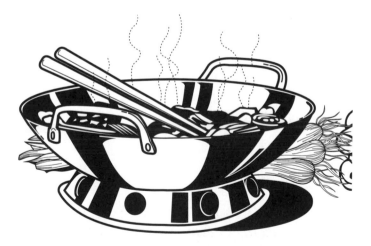

Spaghetti Squash Tarragon

Cholesterol Free
Wheat/Gluten Free
Milk/Casein Free
Egg Free
Suitable through Stage IV

This is a delicious vegetable dish that can be served alone or with rice. It is a great alternative to pasta. The dish has a sweet and savory taste. Begin cooking the garbanzo beans several hours in advance, then start the remainder of the recipe at least an hour and a half before you plan to serve.

1 large or 2 small spaghetti squash

1-1/2 c. dry garbanzo beans, cooked according to directions in *Mainly Beans*

2 medium leeks

4 T. expeller pressed safflower oil

2 tsp. sea salt

1 tsp. dried tarragon

1/2 tsp. celery seed

1 chopped fresh tomato (optional)

1 c. water

Cut the squash in half, preferably lengthwise. Scoop out seeds and the obviously stringy pulp (the edible part of the squash is less stringy). *Cook the squash:* **Stovetop directions:** place open side down into 2" water, cover, and boil until inside is soft. **Oven Directions:** place open side down on a greased cookie sheet. Bake at 350F for about 45 minutes. **Microwave directions:** microwave whole squash on "high" in a small amount of water for 7-10 minutes. *Continue*: When squash is soft,

scoop out the fleshy part of the squash, separating it from the shell. This part will resemble spaghetti. ***Slice*** the leeks and ***saute*** in oil. Add spaghetti squash, tomatoes (optional) and seasonings. Add garbanzos and water. Simmer about 15 minutes, covered. Serve hot.

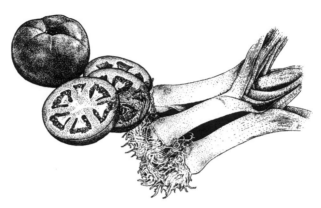

Zucchini Surprise

Milk/Casein Free
Suitable through Stage II

Like many good things in life, this started out as a mistake. It has a pudding-like consistency and kids love it.

> 1/3 c. unprocessed clover honey
>
> 1/2 c. butter
>
> 1 egg
>
> 2 small or one large zucchini
>
> 1-1/2 c. whole wheat flour

Puree everything together in blender or food processor. Bake at 350F for a cooked pudding, or fry it for a sweet pancake. Serve hot.

Vegetable Herb Souffle

Milk/Casein Free
Suitable through Stage II

This casserole souffle tastes like an over stuffed omelette, and is great to serve to company.

6 large eggs

4-5 medium zucchini, grated

4-5 large carrots, peeled and grated

1 large stalk broccoli, chopped into small pieces

3/4 c. whole wheat matzah meal (optional)

1-2 tsp. sea salt

1 tsp. dried basil

1 tsp. dried marjoram

1 tsp. dried thyme

Preheat the oven to 325F. **Separate** five of the six eggs, placing both yolks and whites into large bowls. Break the sixth egg into the yolks. Mix the yolks and set aside. **Add** the vegetables to the egg yolk mixture. Mix. Add matzah meal (optional), salt to taste and herbs. Mix well. The mixture will be very watery. **Beat** the egg whites with an electric mixer on high until stiff peaks form. Fold the whites into the vegetable mixture. Pour into an oiled 9x13 pyrex baking pan. **Bake** at 325F for about an hour. Serve piping hot.

Acorn Squash Kugel

Milk/Casein Free
Suitable through Stage II

This is a "passed around" recipe that has been modified for a yeast-free diet. Everyone loves this pudding. Eliminate the cinnamon if it's a problem for you.

2 whole acorn squash

1/2 c. whole wheat flour

1/3 - 1/2 c. clover honey

3 eggs

1 stick unsalted butter (1/2 c.), melted

1/2 tsp. cinnamon

Preheat oven to 350F. Cook acorn squash by putting one at a time, whole, in microwave for 12 minutes on "high."   Cool to about room temperature. *Cut* squash in half. Scoop out and discard the seeds. Scoop out pulp and put in a large bowl. *Mash* well with a fork or potato masher. Add remaining ingredients and mix well. *Bake* uncovered in a greased, 9x9 baking pan or 1-1/2 quart casserole dish at 350F degrees for one hour. The kugel will rise, then fall when you take it out. Don't be alarmed. Cool before serving.

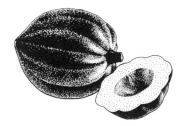

Spinach Kugel

Milk/Casein Free
Wheat/Gluten Free
Suitable through Stage IV

This is a type of spinach pudding (kugel) for spinach lovers, perhaps the most controversial recipe in this cookbook! I have included the recipe because we love it, even though not everybody does. You can serve this hot or cold. Take out the spinach to defrost several hours before you begin cooking this dish. We do not recommend fresh spinach, as it changes the consistency completely.

    4 pkgs. (10-oz.) frozen chopped spinach

    4 eggs

    1 tsp. sea salt

    1/2 to 1 tsp. dried basil

    1/2 to 1 tsp. dried oregano

    1/2 tsp. tarragon (optional)

    1 T. expeller pressed safflower oil

Defrost the frozen spinach in a microwave on "low" setting or on the counter top, if you have time. Drain off as much water as possible, without wringing out the spinach. *Preheat* the oven to 350F. *Mix* the spinach to break up lumps, then mix in the eggs, seasonings and oil. If you prefer less highly seasoned casseroles, use the lower amount of herbs. *Bake* in an oiled casserole dish (2 qt.) uncovered for 1 to 1-1/2 hours at 350F, until the casserole is set.

Stir-Fried Chinese Cabbage or Bok Choy

> *Cholesterol Free*
> *Wheat/Gluten Free*
> *Milk/Casein Free*
> *Egg Free*
> *Suitable through Stage IV*

1 large head of Napa (Chinese) Cabbage *or* 1 large bunch bok choy (white stemmed variety) *or* several small bunches of baby bok choy (green stemmed variety)

expeller pressed safflower oil, for frying

sea salt, to taste

1 tsp. minced garlic (optional)

1 tsp. minced fresh ginger root (optional)

Prepare the cabbage by cutting off the bottom inch, which contains a lot of the dirt. Separate each leaf and wash individually. Remove any brown parts. Place washed leaves in a colander and rinse again. Chop into pieces about 1 inch wide. If the leaves are large, slice down the center of the stem. Drain in the colander. *Heat a wok* on high. Place about 2 T. of oil in the bottom of the wok; heat, but don't smoke the oil. When oil is hot, add the cabbage all at once. *Sprinkle* 1/2 tsp. of sea salt over the cabbage. *Stir fry* by pushing cabbage up against side, pulling more down into the bottom of the wok, and turning over and over. The cabbage will steam. You can put a cover on the wok to speed up the cooking. When cabbage is very soft, it is done. Check your seasonings. If desired, *add* ginger and garlic and cook a minute longer. Tastes great served over **Basic Brown Rice** or **Fluffy Rice.**

Toasted Eggplant and Zucchini Casserole

> *Wheat/Gluten Free (using rice pasta)*
> *Milk/Casein Free*
> *Suitable through Stage IV*

This is a very different tasting casserole with an Italian flavor. It takes some time to prepare, but is not difficult.

For recipe containing wheat: 6 oz. whole wheat noodles

For Wheat/Gluten Free recipe: 10 oz. Pastariso rice pasta

6 medium zucchini

2 small eggplants

2 tsp. dried basil or 6 tsp. fresh chopped basil, plus more to taste

2 large cloves garlic

3 jumbo or 4 large eggs

1 bunch scallions, chopped

expeller pressed safflower oil

canola or safflower oil cooking spray (optional)

sea salt to taste

Cook the noodles according to package directions and set them aside. Prepare the vegetables while the noodles are cooking.
Begin toasting the vegetables while the noodles are cooking.
Peel and thinly slice the eggplant. If the eggplants are large, cut them in half before slicing so the slices are a more manageable size. Using an electric skillet on highest heat, *pour* a very small

amount of safflower oil into the skillet. Use a paper towel to rub it around. *Lay several slices* of eggplant on the skillet and let them cook for several minutes until the skillet side is toasted brown. *Turn* them over and continue to cook until the other side is brown. They should be tender. Remove those slices and set them aside. *Continue to cook* all the eggplant in this manner. *While the eggplant is cooking*, slice the zucchini into thin slices and toast in the same manner you did the eggplant. While the zucchini is cooking, *chop* the scallions into small pieces and mince the garlic. *Oil* or spray a 9x9 inch pyrex casserole dish, or a 7x11 inch pyrex pan. When the vegetables are done, *place* a layer of eggplant on the bottom of the pan. *Sprinkle* with some of the basil, garlic, scallions and salt. Place a layer of noodles over the herbs. Then layer some zucchini, sprinkling with basil, garlic, scallions and salt. Place a layer of noodles over that. *Continue layering* until all ingredients are used. If you run out of herbs, you may add more, so there are herbs in each layer. *Beat* the eggs in a bowl. Gently pour them over the casserole, using a fork to poke holes in the layers so the egg drifts through. *Bake* uncovered at 350F degrees for 50 minutes, or until the egg sets.

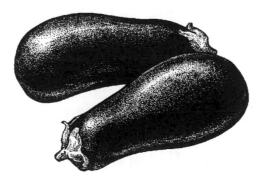

Zesty Eggplant Relish

Cholesterol Free
Wheat/Gluten Free
Milk/Casein Free
Egg Free
Suitable through Stage IV

This dish is an excellent make-ahead dish. It is better cold than hot, and the flavors of the eggplant and garlic can mingle. This recipe takes at least an hour to make, including the time to bake the eggplant. It's a good recipe to make when you have other foods to bake at the same time.

Canola or safflower oil no-stick cooking spray, or extra expeller pressed safflower oil

2 large, firm eggplants

2 cloves garlic, finely chopped

4 T. expeller pressed safflower oil

1/2 tsp. sea salt, or salt to taste

Preheat oven to 350F. Spray a cookie sheet with canola oil spray or lightly grease with safflower oil. *Wash* the eggplants and place them on the cookie sheet. Bake for about 1 hour, until the eggplants puff up, the peel is crisp, and the eggplant soft inside. If you prick the skin, the eggplant will deflate and be soft and mushy. *Cool* until you can handle easily. Peel the eggplant by scooping out the insides. Now chop the garlic. Using a fork or pastry blender or two knives, *mash* the pulp with the chopped garlic. Add salt and oil. The longer this sits, the better it tastes. It's a good dish to make the day before you serve it. Keeps for two days in the refrigerator.

Eggplant Tomato Relish

Cholesterol Free
Wheat/Gluten Free
Milk/Casein Free
Egg Free
Suitable through Stage IV

This is a variation on *Zesty Eggplant*. Tasting better cold than hot, this is also a good make-ahead dish. Start baking the eggplant an hour before you will mix in the tomatoes.

canola or safflower oil no-stick cooking spray, or extra expeller pressed safflower oil

2 medium-sized eggplants

1 c. home-canned tomatoes *or* 1 large fresh tomato, peeled and chopped

sea salt to taste

Preheat the oven to 350F. Spray a cooking sheet with no-stick cooking spray or lightly grease with safflower oil. *Wash* the eggplants and place them, whole, on the cookie sheet. *Bake* at 350F for about an hour, or until they are very soft inside. Check the eggplants after half an hour and turn them if they are burning. Remove from oven and cool until you can handle them. *Scrape* the insides out of the peel and place in a medium-sized bowl. *Mash* or chop until the pieces are very small. *Add* tomatoes. If using canned tomatoes, use juice, too. Add salt to taste.

Carrot Tzimmes

Cholesterol Free
Wheat/Gluten Free
Milk/Casein Free
Egg Free
Suitable through Stage IV

Everyone loves a "tzimmes" (pronounced tsimmus) which is like a very sweet fruit stew.

4 large carrots

4 pitted prunes

1 pear

1 large or 2 medium yams

juice of one fresh lemon

1 c. water, plus more

Preheat oven to 350F. *Peel and chop* the carrots into one inch chunks. *Chop* the prunes into small pieces. *Peel and chop* the pear into small chunks. *Peel and cube* the yams into large cubes, one to two inches. *Mix* all ingredients together in a covered casserole dish. *Bake* at 350F for at least an hour. Check water periodically to make sure the casserole is moist. Add water if necessary. The longer it bakes, the better it tastes.

Baked Winter Squash or Pumpkin

> *Wheat/Gluten Free*
> *Milk/Casein Free (with butter)*
> *Egg Free*
> *Suitable through Stage IV*

Baked winter squash is a delight on a fall or winter evening. This is a recipe that you make using your own judgment, what my grandmother used to call "by the feel." It can't turn out wrong. Try it!

Any amount winter squash (butternut, hubbard, pumpkin, acorn)

small amount of expeller pressed safflower oil

butter to taste (optional)

unprocessed clover honey to taste

Preheat the oven to 375F. While the oven is heating, *cut* the squash in half and scoop out the seeds and the stringy pulp. If desired, save the large seeds to roast according to directions in *Roasted Pumpkin Seeds*. *Cut* the squash into manageable chunks that will fit nicely in a corning ware or pyrex baking pan or casserole dish. Leave the peel on. *Lightly oil* your baking dish with the safflower oil to prevent sticking. Place the squash, pulp side up, in the baking dish. The fit should be tight. Put a thin pat of butter on each piece. *Drizzle* honey generously over the squash. *Cover* tightly with a casserole lid or aluminum foil. *Bake* at 375F for 60 minutes or more until the squash is very soft. Remove from the oven and enjoy now or later. Scoop the squash out of the skin and serve with the sauce that is in your baking dish.

Garden Lasagna

> Cholesterol Free
> Wheat/Gluten Free
> Milk/Casein Free (with butter)
> Egg Free
> Suitable through Stage IV

Lasagna on a yeast free, Wheat/Gluten Free and Milk/Casein Free diet? Absolutely! This recipe makes enough lasagna to fit in one deep 9x13 inch lasagna pan, **or** one standard 9x13 inch pyrex pan, plus one 8x8 inch casserole dish. It tastes better the second day, so it's a good make ahead dish. Because this recipe requires a significant amount of time to prepare, start early in the day. The effort is more than worth while. In addition to the preparation time for precooking the vegetables, allow one hour to bake, plus half an hour to cool.

Sauce

32 plum tomatoes

1-1/2 T. dried basil

1-1/2 T. dried oregano

3 T. butter

3 T. sea salt

water as needed

Begin making the sauce early in the day, or even the night before. The longer this cooks, the better it will taste. *Chop* the tomatoes and set aside. *Melt* the butter in a large skillet and heat until it sizzles. *Add* the tomatoes and mix. *Add* the seasonings. Cover and simmer for several hours. Add water if necessary to prevent sticking and to thin out the sauce.

Filling:

2 10-oz. packages rice lasagna noodles (Pastariso brand)

1 large bunch broccoli

2 large bunches of spinach (about 10 oz. each)

2-4 medium zucchini

6 T. butter

1/4 red bell pepper

1 green bell pepper

1 large tomato

1 c. cooked kidney, anasazi or navy beans

1-3 T. sea salt

1-3 T. dried basil

1-3 T. dried oregano

1-2 c. water

expeller pressed safflower oil or cooking spray for oiling pans

Prepare the noodles according to package directions, if using cooked noodles. For additional directions using uncooked noodles, see note at end. When the noodles are cooked, cool to room temperature. ***Chop*** the broccoli into very small pieces. Set aside. Thoroughly clean and ***chop*** the spinach into very small pieces. Set aside. ***Slice*** the zucchini thinly and set aside. ***Cook the vegetables:*** Melt 2 T. butter in a large skillet. ***Saute*** the broccoli just until tender. Remove and set aside. Melt another 2 T. butter in the skillet. ***Saute*** the spinach until bright and tender. Remove and set aside. Drain the juice. Melt another 2 T. butter in the skillet. ***Saute*** the zucchini until bright and tender. Remove and set aside. ***Chop*** the bell peppers and the tomato. Set aside.

Assembly Instructions Continued on Next Page. . .

To assemble the lasagna: Preheat the oven to 375F. Lightly oil or spray a pyrex lasagna pan. Have all of the vegetables handy, as well as a few tablespoonsful each of basil, oregano and sea salt. Start by thinning the sauce with 1 c. of water. You now will place all of the ingredients in the pan in lawyers: sauce, noodles, beans, vegetables, herbs, then repeat: sauce, noodles, beans, vegetables, herbs and salt, and so on. To do this: *Spread* some sauce on the bottom of a pyrex lasagna pan. *Place a layer* of noodles on the sauce. *Sprinkle* 1/2 of the beans, as well as 1/2 of each of the vegetables, including the peppers and tomatoes, on the noodles. Generously sprinkle basil, oregano and salt over the vegetables. Cover the whole layer generously with sauce. *Spread another* layer of noodles over the sauce and repeat the first layer. For the final layer, spread a layer of noodles over the previous layer. Spread the rest of the sauce generously over the noodles. *Oil or spray* a large sheet of aluminum foil. *Cover* the pan very tightly with the foil, greased side down. If you do not wish to use foil, substitute an oven bag, just spread over the top. *Bake at 375F* for one hour. Remove from oven. Preferably, let *cool* to room temperature, then refrigerate covered overnight. Reheat, then cut and serve. If serving the same day, allow to cool at least 60 minutes before cutting. Serve warm.

Additional directions for using uncooked needles:

If you choose to use uncooked noodles, the top layer will turn out very crunchy. You will need to add one cup of water after assembling the lasagna, before baking, and add additional water during baking. The lasagna needs to bake about 15 minutes longer.

Roasted Pumpkin Seeds

Cholesterol Free
Wheat/Gluten Free
Milk/Casein Free
Egg Free
Suitable through Stage IV

What better snack than fresh roasted pumpkin seeds? If you have any left over, you can save them in an airtight container and snack on them when you want.

> Fresh seeds from a pumpkin or large winter squash
>
> sea salt to taste

Wash the seeds thoroughly, separating them from the stringy pulp. Try to remove as much pulp as possible. *Spread* out the wet seeds in a single layer on an ungreased cookie sheet. A few strands of fiber may remain attached to them, which is not harmful. Sprinkle the seeds liberally with sea salt. *For quick roasting,* preheat the oven to 350F and place the cookie sheet in the oven. Bake for an hour, checking the seeds every 20 minutes and stirring them around to prevent sticking. Remove from the oven when the seeds are crispy, browned and puffy. *For slow roasting*, preheat the oven to 250F. Place the cookie sheet in the oven for several hours or overnight, until the seeds are roasted dry and browned. *Storage and serving* : Let the seeds cool to room temperature. Serve immediately, or store in an airtight container. Pumpkin seeds can be eaten with the shell, or you can crack the shells and just eat the seeds.

Ratatouille

> *Cholesterol Free*
> *Wheat/Gluten Free*
> *Milk/Casein Free*
> *Egg Free*
> *Suitable through Stage IV*

Ratatouille is a layered Mediterranean dish, the basic ingredients of which are eggplant, garlic and onion. Because you can make endless variations of this dish, I give only the basic instructions. Leave the rest to your imagination! This stove top recipe tastes great made in advance. Allow at least two hours for the flavors to be absorbed. Serve with **Basic Brown Rice** mixed into the Ratatouille. This recipe makes enough to serve 6 very hungry people. For less, decrease the ingredients proportionately.

2 whole eggplants

6 medium zucchini

1 bunch scallions or two medium leeks

4 cloves garlic

8-10 tomatoes

2 T. expeller pressed safflower oil

3 tsp. dried basil

3 tsp. dried oregano

3 tsp. dried dill

1 T. sea salt, plus more to taste

Begin *heating* a 6-quart pot on low. While the pot is heating, *prepare the ingredients.* First, you will chop or slice the ingredients. Then you will layer them, similar to lasagna (but without the noodles!). The key to success is staying organized.

To begin, get out four plates and a few small bowls. Then begin preparing the vegetables. ***Cut the eggplants*** in half lengthwise and slice them into one quarter inch thick slices crosswise, leaving the peels on. You will have half moon shapes. Discard the tough ends. Put the eggplant slices on a place. Next, ***slice*** the zucchini into quarter inch thick rounds and place them on another plate. Chop the scallions or leeks and place in a small bowl. ***Chop*** the garlic and place in a small bowl. ***Slice*** the tomatoes into one quarter inch thick slices and place on a plate. Have the herbs and salt ready. ***Pour the oil*** into the kettle and heat, to prevent the first layer from sticking. When the oil is hot, ***begin layering*** the ingredients, sprinkling small amount of herbs and salt after every few layers. For example, place a layer of zucchini, then scallions and some garlic, then eggplant, then sprinkle herbs and salt. Layer tomatoes, then zucchini, then more herbs and salt, etc. There is no incorrect way to do this, as long as you space out your layers so everything is used and cooks evenly. Don't worry if you have a pot heaped high with vegetables. They cook down to about half the bulk. When all ingredients are used up, ***cover***, turn the heat up to low/medium. Bring to a slow boil, then reduce to simmer. Cook for at least 30 minutes, until the eggplant is done. This tastes best if simmered for about 2 hours, to allow the flavors to seep through all the vegetables.

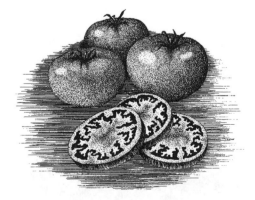

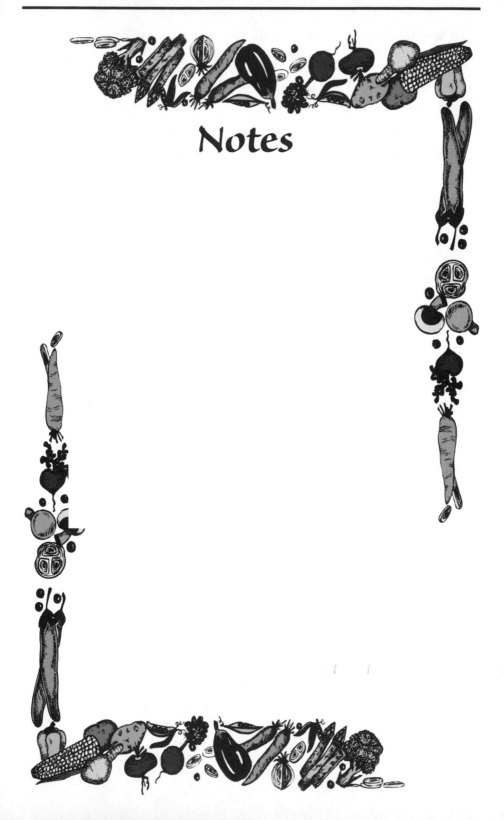

Notes

Mainly Meat, Fish & Poultry

Yeast free diets work best with very limited meat, poultry and fish. At times, though, some animal protein tastes good and is fun for a change of pace and to ensure an adequate supply of Vitamin B-12. We have included only a few easy to make recipes for basic fish and chicken, and a handful of recipes for the meats of choice, veal and lamb. You can use the principles in these recipes to expand your personal repertoire.

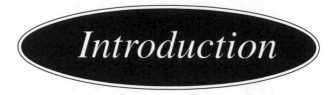

Introduction

Yeast free diets work best with very limited meat, poultry and fish. This statement will startle people who have gone on other yeast free diets. Many of those diets are very high in animal protein and low in carbohydrate.

The reason for this is that Dr. Orian Truss, who first published the idea that the yeast *Candida Albicans* can cause health problems in *The Missing Diagnosis*, observed that yeast grow well in carbohydrate and not particularly well in protein. Therefore, he reasoned, one should remove carbohydrate from the diet so the yeast doesn't grow as well. Subsequently, the standard anti-yeast diet recommends eliminating all sugar and yeast from bread and adding more meat and fish.

In my practice, I have found that this diet is not optimal, for reasons I explain in an earlier chapter, ***The Story Behind the Book***. Many of my patients have followed the standard yeast free diet, but have enjoyed few results. The reason for their lack of results is not their lack of effort, but the fact that the main dietary yeast offenders (vinegar and barley malt) had been left in their diets. In fact, most of the anti-yeast and allergy related cookbooks have vinegar as a staple food and recommend a diet high in animal protein, which is problematic, and nuts, which are thoroughly mold contaminated. My experience with my other patients is that this recommendation of using meat and eliminating almost all carbohydrate is wrong.

When yeast spoils meat, the toxic chemicals formed are worse than those formed by yeast in carbohydrate. In addition, chicken and pigs are fed cottonseed meal which is contaminated with a fungus called Aspergillus. I speculate that the animals store the Aspergillus poisons in their fat . This technique is a common way for animals to handle poisons. It is possible that storing the fungus poisons is one reason why yeast sensitive patients should not eat large amounts of meat.

Notwithstanding these comments, meat from the right sources and in small quantities is acceptable on the anti-yeast diet. Some animal protein is important for people to feel they have not completely given up their previous life, and also to ensure adequate supplies of Vitamin B-12. If you are on a diet that eliminates not only yeast, but casein (dairy) and eggs, you have no animal sources of protein left and may run into Vitamin B-12 deficiencies unless you take supplements or eat meat every once in awhile. We cannot make our own vitamin B-12 from plant sources.

If you do choose to eat meat, we recommend eating more meat than fish or poultry, and using veal or lamb as a meat source. At Stage IV, we recommend eliminating fish and greatly restricting poultry to a small amount every once in awhile. Veal and lamb are the easiest meat to digest for extremely sensitive people.

For stages I through III, we recommend using very fresh, mild fish, such as filet of sole, and very fresh poultry that has not been feed antibiotics or hormones. At least one brand of Kosher poultry (Empire) and some "organic" meats advertise that their products have not been fed antibiotics.

The recipes in this book are very basic. You can use these recipes as guidelines to develop your own recipes at home.

So, start here and have some fun learning new ways to cook your old favorites.

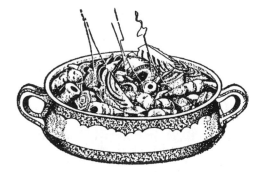

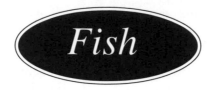

Lemon Baked Fish Fillets

> *Wheat/Gluten Free*
> *Milk/Casein Free*
> *Egg Free*
> *Suitable through Stage III*

This recipe is simple and pleasing, and can be used for any kind of fish that you tolerate.

1-1/2 lbs. fresh fish fillets from a mild fish, such as fillet of sole

expeller pressed safflower oil or nonstick cooking spray

sea salt to taste

1 fresh lemon

1 clove fresh garlic

Preheat the oven to 350F. *Lightly grease* a pyrex or corning wear casserole dish, or a 7x11 inch pyrex pan, with safflower oil or cooking spray. *Wash* the fish thoroughly. Salt the fillets lightly on both sides. Lay the fish in the casserole dish or pan. Squeeze the entire lemon over the fish. Chop the garlic and sprinkle it over the fish. Cover. Place in oven. Cook until the fish flakes, but does not fall apart, 15 minutes to 40 minutes, depending on the thickness of your fillets. Serve with any rice or pasta dish and a salad with *Creamy Cucumber Dressing*.

Pan Fried Fish

Wheat/Gluten Free
Milk/Casein Free
Egg Free
Suitable through Stage III

Fried fish is a little perkier than baked fish, but has lots more fat and calories. Kids like this recipe. Use this recipe for just about any fish you enjoy eating, that you tolerate.

1-1/2 lbs. fresh fish fillets of a mild fish, such as fillet of sole

2 T. butter, plus more if desired

sea salt to taste

1 fresh lemon

2 cloves fresh garlic

expeller pressed safflower oil, if desired.

Heat a large, heavy frying pan on low heat, or an electric frying pan set to the first or second setting. *Melt* the butter in the frying pan. Wash the fish thoroughly. Salt the fillets lightly on both sides. Turn the heat to medium-high so the butter sizzles, but does not smoke. *Lay the fillets* in the frying pan. Squeeze the entire lemon over the fish. Chop the garlic and sprinkle it over the fish. As the fish cooks, add more butter or oil if necessary to prevent sticking (especially in a cast iron pan). *Cook* until the fish is light brown on one side, then turn over. Cook until the fish flakes, but does not fall apart.

Gefilte Fish

> *Traditional*:
> *Milk/Casein Free*
> *Suitable through Stage II*
>
> *Simplified*:
> *Wheat/Gluten Free*
> *Milk/Casein Free*
> *Egg Free*
> *Suitable through Stage IV*

Cooking Notes--Recipes follow on next two pages!

I love gefilte fish (pronounced ga-fill-ta), which is a traditional Eastern-European Jewish dish. It literally means "stuffed fish." Over time, the stuffing has become the dish. Homemade gefilte fish is very easy, and takes less than half an hour to prepare from the time the fish is ground or chopped.

The key to success in making gefilte fish for a yeast-free diet is using extremely fresh fish. Take the fish home immediately from the market and do not let it sit out. Prepare it within an hour or two, but refrigerate if you delay even a few minutes! Fish begins to spoil very quickly and produces toxins that are hard for yeast sensitive people to handle. Made this way, the fish has a light and appealing flavor.

The traditional recipe contains both gluten and eggs in the fish balls; **the simplified recipe** has no gluten or eggs. One way to cook this recipe is to divide the broth into two pots, then remove a portion of the fish mixture before adding the eggs and matzah meal, and continue with the other mixture to add the matzah meal and egg. This way, you will have a partial recipe of *Traditional Gefilte Fish* and a partial recipe of *Simplified Gefilte Fish*.

The complete recipe makes enough gefilte fish for about 8-10 very hungry people.

See next pages for the recipe!

Broth for both recipes of Gefilte Fish:

2-3 carrots

1 fresh (with green tops) Spanish onion *or* 2 large leeks *or* 1 bunch scallions

4 stalks celery

2 tsp. sea salt

1/2 tsp. pepper

2 qt. water, to start

Peel and chop the carrots. Chop the onions. Chop the celery. Place all ingredients in a 4-quart stock pot. Cover; bring to boil, then reduce to simmer. Cook for 20 minutes while you are preparing the fish.

Fish for Traditional Gefilte Fish:

2 lb. fish fillets of any combination you like, including whitefish, pike, "buffalo fish" or other white- or yellow-fleshed fish

> Note: you may have the fish ground at a fish market, to save time

1/2 c. whole wheat or white matzah meal

1 T. sea salt

1/4 tsp. pepper

2-3 T. chopped fresh parsley (or more, to taste)

1-2 eggs

Continued on next pages!

If not using pre-ground fish, wash the fish thoroughly, then grind it in a meat grinder or chop it very fine using a sharp cleaver. *Chopping* the fish takes about 10 minutes of fast, steady work and is a great way to release tension! *Mix* the fish with the matzah meal, 1 T. salt, 1/4 tsp. pepper, chopped parsley and 1 egg. The mixture should be pretty stiff and sticky. Add the second egg if the fish mixture is too stiff or dry. If the mixture is too loose and will not form into balls, add more matzah meal. *Form* the fish into small balls or cakes about 2 inches in diameter. Be sure to press the fish balls together, or they will disintegrate during cooking.   Place gently with a spoon into the simmering stock. Bring the stock to boil again, then reduce to a gentle rolling boil. *Cook* for 20 min. Add more water to cover fish, as needed.

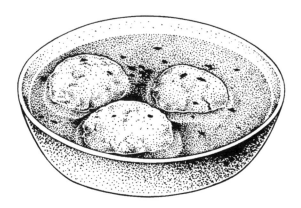

Fish for Simplified Gefilte Fish:

2 lb. fish fillets of any combination you like, including whitefish, pike, "buffalo fish" or other white- or yellow-fleshed fish

> Note: for convenience, you may have this ground at a fish market.

1 T. sea salt

1/4 tsp. pepper

2-3 T. chopped fresh parsley (or more, to taste)

If not using pre-ground fish, wash the fish thoroughly, then grind it in a meat grinder or chop it very fine using a sharp cleaver. *Chopping* the fish takes about 10 minutes of fast, steady work and is a great way to release tension! *Mix* in the sea salt, pepper, and the chopped parsley. This mixture will be fairly wet and may seem to fall apart. *Form the fish* into small balls or cakes about 2 inches in diameter. Be sure to press the fish balls together, or they will disintegrate during cooking. *Place* gently with a spoon into the simmering stock. Bring the stock to boil again, then reduce to a gentle rolling boil. Cook for 20 min. Add more water to cover fish, as needed. Serve hot or cold.

Basic Tuna Salad

Wheat/Gluten Free
Milk/Casein Free
Egg Free
Suitable through Stage III

Tuna salad is such a staple that many people find giving up mayonnaise almost beyond consideration. You can make a deliciously light tuna salad with just a few ingredients. Many nonsensitive people even prefer this salad to traditional mayonnaise based tuna salad.

To make tuna salad, start with canned tuna packed only in distilled water. This usually is labelled sodium free or low-sodium. "Tuna packed in water" is not acceptable, because the water contains many additives, including the mysterious "vegetable broth." Sometimes "tuna packed in water" contains casein.

Serve with any rice, or pasta dish, or as a side salad with *Egg Salad* and *Parsley Potato Salad*. Or, just eat it plain or on *Delicious and Nutritious Whole Wheat Bread.*

1 6-oz. can sodium free or low sodium tuna (white or chunk light)

1/4 tsp. dried dill (optional)

1/2 tsp. sea salt

1 T. expeller pressed safflower oil

1/2 T. water (optional), plus more for taste

chopped celery (optional)

Empty the can of tuna into a bowl. Fork-chop it until the tuna is the desired consistency. Everyone's taste differs! Mix in the dill (if desired) and salt. Add the oil; mix thoroughly. Add the water if you desire a wetter consistency. You may add more water if you wish. Add chopped celery. Serve!

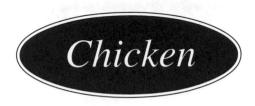

Roasted Chicken with Herbs

> *Wheat/Gluten Free*
> *Milk/Casein Free*
> *Egg Free*
> *Suitable through Stage III*

This recipe takes about five minutes to assemble, using chicken pieces, and tastes like a dream. This is a "by the feel" recipe that will turn out differently for each cook, but taste equally delicious.

expeller pressed safflower oil

sea salt, to taste

1 large fryer chicken (about 4 lbs.), cut into pieces

several pinches of fresh or dried dill

several pinches of fresh or dried marjoram

Lightly oil a shallow baking pan. *Salt* the chicken pieces, then lay them in the pan. Lightly rub oil onto each piece. Generously *sprinkle* dill and marjoram onto each piece of chicken. *Bake* at 375F for one hour, or until the juices run clear.

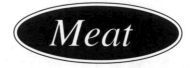

Veal Stew

> *Wheat/Gluten Free*
> *Milk/Casein Free*
> *Egg Free*
> *Suitable through Stage IV*

Start this recipe early in the day. The longer it cooks, the more tender the meat and more flavorful the stew. Serve over pasta or *Basic Brown Rice.*

4 medium zucchini

7 medium red potatoes

10-12 plum tomatoes

4 T. expeller pressed safflower oil

2 lb. veal stew meat

1 T. dried basil

1 T. dried oregano

1 T. sea salt

6 c. water

Slice the zucchini into thin slices. Set aside. Peel the potatoes and cube them into 1/2 inch cubes. Set aside. Chop the tomatoes into large pieces. Set aside. *Heat* the oil in the bottom of a large stock pot. If your meat is not cut into chunks, wash it and cut it. When the oil is hot, *add the stew meat* to brown. When it is browned, add the sliced zucchini. Saute until zucchini is soft. *Add* the tomatoes, potatoes, herbs, salt and water. Bring to a boil. Reduce to simmer. Let this cook for 2-3 hours before serving. If necessary, add more water. Test salt before serving and add more if necessary. Serve over rice or rice noodles.

Stir-Fried Veal

Wheat/Gluten Free
Milk/Casein Free
Egg Free
Suitable through Stage IV

4 medium zucchini

2 tomatoes

3 stalks broccoli

5 stalks celery

1 lb. ground veal *or* 1 lb. thinly sliced veal meat , plus 1/2 tsp. each sea salt oregano, basil and dill

1 tsp. each dried oregano, basil and dill

sea salt to taste

2-4 T. expeller pressed safflower oil, plus more to taste

1 c. water

Slice the zucchini, *chop* the tomatoes and broccoli, and *slice* the celery into thin slices and set all aside. *Brown* the ground veal, adding extra herbs, or brown the veal slices in a small amount of safflower oil.   Remove and set aside. If necessary, add 1 T. more oil. *Add* the zucchini and stir fry until it is soft. *Sprinkle* a pinch of sea salt over it while cooking. Remove and set aside. *Repeat* with the broccoli, then the celery, cooking each vegetable separately, adding more oil as necessary. Then *cook* the tomatoes until they form a sauce. *Add* the herbs to the tomatoes. *Add* all of the other cooked vegetables and the meat and stir thoroughly. Add water at the very end, to form a sauce.   For best texture, serve within about 5 minutes, enough time to allow the food to absorb flavor. Serve over *Basic Brown Rice*.

Extra Garlic Spaghetti Sauce and Meatballs

Wheat/Gluten Free
Milk/Casein Free
Egg Free
Suitable through Stage IV

If you like Italian food, you'll love this. This is similar to *Spaghetti Sauce and Meatballs*, but uses lots of extra garlic and more oregano. This recipe also uses more meat for the volume of sauce, so it is a little richer. Serve over whole wheat or rice pasta.

Sauce:

14 medium tomatoes

6 cloves garlic

2 T. expeller pressed safflower oil

1 T. dried basil

2 T. dried oregano

1/2 T. sea salt, or salt to taste

Chop the tomatoes and set aside. Mince the garlic. Heat the oil in a large pot. When hot, add the garlic and saute. *Add* the tomatoes, basil, oregano and salt. Cook until the tomatoes are very soft and saucy. *While the sauce* is cooking, make the meatballs, then continue: *Cool* to a manageable temperature, then *puree* in a blender or food processor until smooth. Put the sauce back in the pot. Heat to a boil, then turn down to a simmer.

Meatballs:

    3 lb. ground veal

    2 tsp. sea salt

    1 T. oregano

    4 T. expeller pressed safflower oil

Mix the veal with the salt and oregano. Form into small meatballs, about one inch in diameter. Press the balls so they do not fall apart during cooking. Heat the oil in a frying pan. When the oil is hot, start browning the meatballs. Turn several times with a fork to be sure they brown all around. When the meatballs are cooked through and brown and crispy on the outside, add them to the sauce. Simmer until serving time.

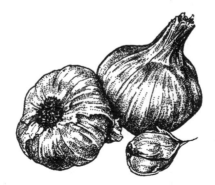

Spaghetti Sauce with Meatballs

> *Wheat/Gluten Free*
> *Milk/Casein Free*
> *Egg Free*
> *Suitable through Stage IV*

This is another rave-review recipe, especially from the kids.

Sauce:

2 T. expeller pressed safflower oil

1 large leek

2 large cloves garlic

1/2 c. fresh oregano leaves, or 2 T. dried oregano

1/2 c. fresh basil leaves, or 2 T. dried basil

1-2 T. sea salt, to taste

20 medium sized tomatoes

Pour the oil into a large pot. Heat on medium high heat. While the oil is heating, *chop* the leek and garlic. Saute them in the hot oil. Add the herbs. *Continue sauteing* until the leeks are tender. *Chop* the tomatoes into large chunks and add to the leek mixture. Add 1 T. sea salt. Bring to a boil; cover; simmer for 30 minutes. Test for salt. *While the sauce* is cooking, make the meatballs, then continue: *Cool* to a manageable temperature. *Puree* the sauce in a blender or food processor. Pour the pureed sauce back in the pot.

Meatballs:

2 lb. ground veal

1 tsp. dried basil

1 tsp. dried oregano

1 tsp. sea salt

2 T. expeller pressed safflower oil

While waiting for the sauce to cook, make the meatballs. *Mix* the veal with the herbs and salt. *Form* into small meatballs about one inch in diameter. Pour the oil into a frying pan and heat it on medium high heat. *Brown* the meatballs in the oil until partially cooked. You will need to turn the meatballs with a fork to get them to brown evenly. Handle these little balls carefully so they won't fall apart!

Gently place the meatballs into the simmering, pureed sauce. Cover; bring to a boil. Reduce to simmer and cook for 30 minutes to an hour. Serve over whole wheat or rice pasta.

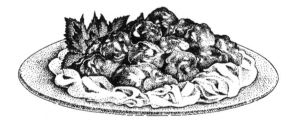

Garden Lasagna with Meat

Wheat/Gluten Free
Milk/Casein Free
Egg Free
Suitable through Stage IV

Lasagna is an all-time favorite. This lasagna is a variation on *Garden Lasagna*. It is a hearty, but not heavy, main dish. Like the *Garden Lasagna*, this is one of the few recipes that is better the second day. If serving the same day, start early! Making the sauce, precooking the vegetables and assembling the lasagna take time. After assembling the lasagna, allow one hour to bake, plus half an hour to cool. You can make this recipe with precooked or uncooked noodles. If using uncooked noodles, be aware that the top layer will turn out very crunchy, but edible. Additional instructions for using uncooked noodles are given at the end of the recipe. We recommend taking the time to precook the noodles. This recipe is designed for one deep 9x13 inch pan of lasagna.

Sauce:

21 plum tomatoes

1 T. dried basil

1 T. dried oregano

2 T. expeller pressed safflower oil

2 T. sea salt

Begin making the sauce early in the day, or even the night before. The longer this cooks, the better it will taste. *Chop* the tomatoes and set aside. *Heat* the oil in a large skillet until it sizzles. *Add* the tomatoes and mix. Add the seasonings. *Cover and simmer* for several hours. *Add* water if necessary to prevent sticking.

Filling:

2 10-oz. packages rice lasagna noodles (Pastariso brand)

1 T. expeller pressed safflower oil

1 lb. ground veal

1 large bunch broccoli, chopped

2-4 medium zucchini, thinly sliced

1 c. cooked kidney, anasazi or navy beans

4 T. expeller pressed safflower oil

1/4 red bell pepper

1 green bell pepper

1 large tomato

1-3 T. each sea salt, dried basil and dried oregano

 1-2 c. water

expeller pressed safflower oil or cooking spray for oiling pans

Precook the noodles according to package directions. When done, cool to room temperature. While the noodles are cooking, *heat a frying* pan on medium. Add the tablespoon of safflower oil. When hot, brown the veal. Set aside. *Heat* 2 T. oil in a large skillet. Saute the broccoli just until tender. Remove and set aside. Heat 2 T. oil in the skillet.   Saute the zucchini until bright and tender. Remove and set aside. *Chop* the bell peppers and the tomato. Set aside.

Assembly Directions on Next Page. . . .

Assembly for Lasagna:

Preheat the oven to 375F. Lightly oil or spray a pyrex lasagna pan. Have all of the vegetables, meat and beans handy, as well as a few tablespoonsful each of basil, oregano and sea salt. You will be assembling the lasagna in two layers consisting of: sauce, noodles, beans, vegetables, meat, herbs. **Thin** the sauce with 1 c. water. Spread some sauce on the bottom of a pyrex lasagna pan. Place a layer of noodles on the sauce. **Sprinkle** 1/2 of the beans, as well as 1/2 of each of the vegetables, including the peppers and tomatoes, on the noodles. Spread half of the meat over the vegetables. **Generously sprinkle** basil, oregano and salt over everything. That ends the first layer. You now will repeat the process! **Cover** the whole layer generously with sauce. **Spread more** noodles over the sauce, then sprinkle the rest of the beans, then the vegetables, meat and tomatoes on the noodles. **Generously sprinkle** basil, oregano and salt over everything. **For the final layer**, spread sauce over the previous layer. Then lay the rest of the noodles over the sauce. **Spread** the rest of the sauce generously over the noodles. **Oil or spray** a large sheet of aluminum foil. **Cover** the pan very tightly with the foil. **Bake** at 375F for one hour. **Remove** from oven. Preferably, let **cool** to room temperature, then refrigerate covered overnight. Reheat, then cut and serve. If serving the same day, allow to cool at least 30 minutes before cutting. Serve warm.

Additional directions for using uncooked needles:

If you use uncooked noodles, the top layer will turn out very crunchy. You will need to add one cup of water after assembling the lasagna, before baking, and add additional water during baking. The lasagna needs to bake about 15 minutes longer.

Veal Meatballs & Potatoes

> *Wheat/Gluten Free*
> *Milk/Casein Free*
> *Egg Free*
> *Suitable through Stage IV*

This is a fun dish to make and serve with children. The longer it cooks, the better it tastes. Serves 6 hungry people.

2 T. expeller pressed safflower oil for sauteing

2 medium zucchini, sliced

2 plum tomatoes, chopped

1 tsp. dried basil

1 tsp. dried oregano

1 T. fresh dill or 1 tsp. dried dill

3/4 tsp. sea salt

4 c. water

4 small red potatoes, peeled and cubed

2 lb. ground veal

1/2 tsp. sea salt

1/2 tsp. dried basil

1/2 tsp. dried oregano

Make the stock: *Heat* a large stock pot on medium-high. *Pour* in the oil for sauteing. Add the zucchini. *Saute* until tender. *Add* the tomatoes, basil, oregano and dill. *Saute* until tomatoes get soft and begin to fall apart. *Add* the water and salt. Bring to a boil; *add* potatoes. Bring to a *boil*; reduce to simmer.
Make the meatballs: *Mix* the ground veal with the herbs and salt. *Tightly form* meat into balls about one inch in diameter. Gently *lower* the meatballs into the simmering stock. The meat is cooked in about 20 minutes, but for more flavor, cook longer.

Lamb Stew

> *Wheat/Gluten Free*
> *Milk/Casein Free*
> *Egg Free*
> *Suitable through Stage IV*

Try this stew for a tasty departure from the ordinary. Start early in the day to allow plenty of time for the stew to stew! Serves 8-10 hungry people.

3 lb. lamb stew meat, including bones, in pieces

water

juice of one fresh lemon

2 T. expeller pressed safflower oil

1 large leek, chopped

5 cloves garlic, minced

6 medium zucchini, sliced

1 T. dried dill weed

1 bay leaf

1-1/2 T. sea salt

5 medium red or white rose potatoes

3 carrots, peeled and chopped (optional)

3 stalks celery, chopped (optional)

Heat a large (6-8 quart) pot. Put the pieces of stew meat in the pot, fat side down, and *braise*, turning every few minutes to keep the meat from burning. Cook until the meat is browned all over, about 20 minutes. *Add* enough water to the pot to fill about half full. Bring to a boil. As the water heats, foam will form on the surface of the water. ***Skim foam*** off. Keep skimming until little to no foam is left. When the foaming stops, add the lemon juice to the lamb. While the lamb is cooking, ***heat*** the oil in a skillet. When oil is hot, add the leek, garlic and zucchini. ***Saute*** them until soft. ***Add to the lamb*** after you have added the lemon juice. ***Add*** the dill, bay leaf and salt. Peel and cube the potatoes into 1/2 inch cubes. Add them to the lamb. If desired, add carrots and celery. ***Add more water*** so the stew comes to within an inch of the top of the pot. Cover. Bring to a boil, then reduce to simmer. ***Cook*** at least two more hours. If desired, remove the lamb from the pot. ***Cool*** until you can handle the lamb, then take the meat off the bones, separate the fat, and put the meat and bones back in the pot. The bones continue to add flavor to the stew, and some people enjoy chewing on them. Although the stew is ready to eat now, you can let it simmer for up to 6 more hours, if desired. The flavors will become even better. Serve hot.

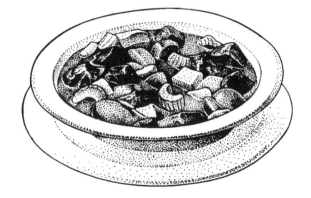

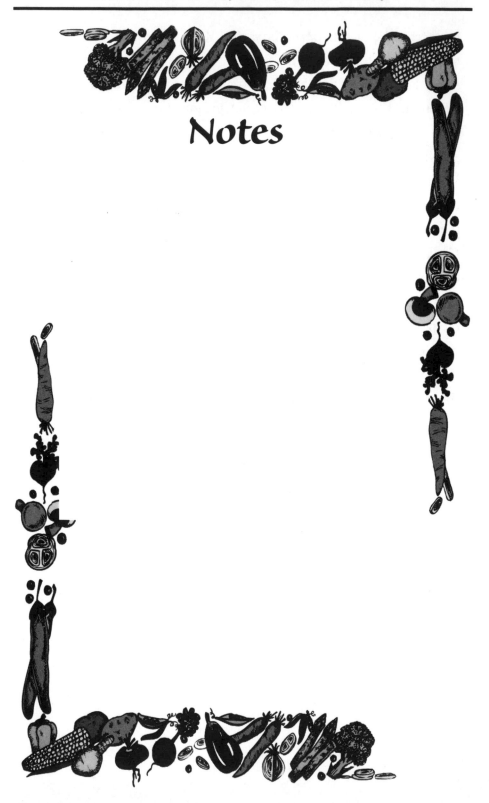

Notes

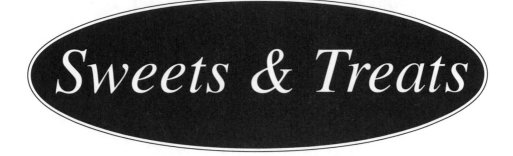

Sweets & Treats

People love sweets and treats, and we have plenty of them! This chapter gives you lots of recipes for:

- *~ Cakes & Dessert Breads*
- *~ Cookies*
- *~ Frostings*
- *~ Pies*
- *~ Candies*
- *~ Sorbets & Ice Milks*
- *~ Sweet Beverages*

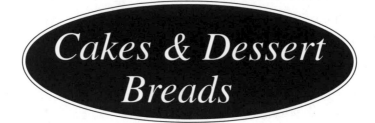

The Best Carrot Cake in the Whole World

Milk/Casein Free
Suitable through Stage II

This recipe is an all-time favorite. The cake is surprisingly light and has great flavor. Use any of the frostings in this book to frost, or just serve plain.

1-1/2 c. expeller pressed safflower oil *or* for more flavor, use 1/2 c. melted unsalted butter and 1 c. safflower oil

1-1/2 c. unprocessed clover honey

4 extra large eggs (for a lighter cake, use 3 eggs)

2-1/2 c. whole wheat pastry flour

2-1/2 tsp. baking powder

1 tsp. baking soda

1 tsp. salt

2 tsp. cinnamon

1 tsp. allspice

2-3 c. grated fresh carrots

Preheat the oven to 350F. Generously grease and flour pans (use either: 2 loaf pans, or one 9x13 inch pan, or a combination of loaf pans, cake pans and muffin cups). In large bowl, **beat** with electric mixer the oil, honey and eggs until well blended. In small bowl, **sift** dry ingredients together. Gradually add dry to wet ingredients, mixing with electric mixer. **Fold in** the carrots by hand. Pour into a 9 x 13 inch pan, or loaf pans, or muffin cups, or two layer pans. **Bake** at 350F until a toothpick comes out dry (about 50-60 minutes for the 9 x 13 pan, 45 minutes for layer pans, 20 minutes for small muffins, 30-35 minutes for loaves). Cool, then frost, if desired.

Variation:

Zucchini Cake

Use one recipe of **The Best Carrot Cake in the Whole World**, but substitute grated zucchini for carrots. After grating the zucchini, place it in a colander and let it sit for 30 minutes, squeezing out the water from time to time. Continue with the cake as in the carrot cake recipe.

Zucchini Bread

Milk/Casein Free (with butter)
Suitable through Stage II

This is lighter than a cake, and not as sweet. The baked cakes freeze well.

  4-5 c. grated zucchini

  1 c. unprocessed clover honey

  1/3 c. melted butter

  2 large eggs

  3 c. whole wheat pastry flour

  1/2 tsp. salt

  1 T. baking powder

  5/8 tsp. allspice

  1 tsp. cinnamon

Preheat the oven to 350F. *Place* the grated zucchini in a colander and stand over a plate or bowl. Set aside. From time to time, press down on the zucchini to eliminate the water that will collect. *Beat* by hand or with an electric mixer the honey, butter, and eggs. In a separate bowl, *mix* the dry ingredients. *Add* the dry to the wet ingredients and mix them in. Press the remaining water out of the zucchini, then *fold* in by hand. Pour the batter into 2 to 3 oiled loaf pans, or make a combination of muffins and loaves. *Bake* loaf cakes at 350F for 35-45 minutes, until a toothpick comes out dry (15 min. for mini-muffins; 20 min. for muffins) The loaves will be fairly heavy. The muffins, especially mini-muffins, come out lighter.

Pumpkin Cake

Milk/Casein Free
Suitable through Stage II

A delicious way to celebrate the fall! Children love this cake. It makes a great Halloween treat to share with schoolmates.

2 c. unprocessed clover honey

1 c. expeller pressed safflower oil

2-1/4 c. pureed fresh pie pumpkin, prepared according to instructions in *A Note on Ingredients*

4 eggs

3 c. whole wheat pastry flour

2 tsp. cinnamon

1/4 tsp. cloves (or 1/2 tsp. allspice)

1/4 tsp. mace

1 T. baking powder

2 tsp. baking soda

1 tsp. salt

Preheat the oven to 325F. Oil 2 ten inch cake pans, or one 9x13 inch pan, or 2 loaf pans, or muffin tins and set aside. *Mix* all ingredients, in order, with an electric mixer. Use the amount of flour that goes with the humidity of the day. 3 cups produces a moist cake on a dry day. If weather is humid, add more flour. *Pour* into well oiled pans or muffin tins. *Bake* at 350F for 45 minutes for a 9x13 inch cake or two loaf pans, or until a toothpick comes out dry (20 minutes for muffins; 35 minutes for mini loaf pans). Freeze any extra cake to enjoy later.

Honey Cake

Milk/Casein Free
Suitable through Stage II

Honey cake is a traditional dessert for the Jewish New Year, symbolizing the sweetness of the New Year. This cake tastes best when made at least a day ahead of time and stored wrapped in aluminum foil and placed in a plastic bag. Freezes well.

4 eggs

1-1/2 c. unprocessed clover honey

1/3 c. expeller pressed safflower oil

1/2 c. water

3 c. whole wheat pastry flour

1/2 tsp. salt

2 tsp. baking powder

1 tsp. baking soda

1/2 tsp. ground cloves

1/2 tsp. ground allspice

Preheat the oven to 325F. *Oil two loaf pans* and set aside. *Separate* the eggs, placing the yolks in a large bowl and the whites in a medium sized bowl. Using an electric mixer, *beat* the yolks with honey until creamy. Add oil and water; beat. *Sift* the dry ingredients, then gradually add to the honey mixture, stirring with a wooden spoon after each addition. *Beat the egg whites* to stiff peaks, then carefully fold them into the batter. Pour into oiled loaf pans. Bake at 325F for 45-60 minutes, until toothpick comes out dry. Allow cake to cool, then wrap in foil and place in a plastic bag.

Cranberry Jewel Bread

Milk/Casein Free
Suitable through Stage II

This bread is very tart, but absolutely delicious for cranberry lovers. It is a perfect light Thanksgiving side dish.

> juice of one freshly squeezed orange, plus water to make one cup
>
> 3 T. expeller pressed safflower oil
>
> 1 c. unprocessed clover honey
>
> 1 egg
>
> 1 tsp. baking powder
>
> 1 tsp. baking soda
>
> 1/2 tsp. salt
>
> 2 c. whole wheat pastry flour
>
> 2-3 c. whole cranberries (one standard size package of fresh cranberries)

Preheat the oven to 350F. Oil two loaf pans and set aside. With an electric mixer, beat the ingredients together, except cranberries, in the order listed. Fold in the cranberries by hand. Pour into oiled loaf pans. Bake at 350F for about 50 minutes, or until a toothpick comes out dry.

Cranberry Apple Bread

Milk/Casein Free
Suitable through Stage I

This bread is beautiful to serve as a light dessert or as part of the main meal. It is very tart and tastes deliciously of cranberries. If you like sweeter breads, follow the alternative directions.

For Tart Bread:

3/4 c. unprocessed clover honey

1 c. water

For Sweeter Bread:

1 c. unprocessed clover honey

3/4 c. water

For all breads:

3-4 medium apples

3 T. expeller pressed safflower oil, plus extra to oil pans

1 egg

1 tsp. baking powder

1 tsp. baking soda

1/2 tsp. salt

2-3/4 c. whole wheat pastry flour + more if necessary

2-3 c. fresh whole cranberries (one standard size package of fresh cranberries)

Preheat the oven to 350F. *Oil* two loaf pans and/or prepare muffin tins. *Peel and chop* the apples and set aside. *Beat* in order with an electric mixer all the ingredients except the cranberries and apples. The batter should be the consistency of a thick cake batter. If it is not, add additional flour. *Fold* in the apples and cranberries. Pour into oiled loaf pans and/or muffin tins. Bake at 350F until a toothpick comes out dry, about 50 minutes for a loaf pan and 30 minutes for muffins.

Apple Honey Bread

> *Milk/Casein Free*
> *Suitable through Stage I*

This bread is sweet and special for the new year.

expeller pressed safflower oil *or* acceptable nonstick cooking spray for greasing pans

3 c. whole wheat pastry flour

4 tsp. baking powder

1 tsp. sea salt

1 egg

1 c. plus 2 T. unprocessed clover honey

1 c. water

1/4 c. expeller pressed safflower oil

2 small apples

Preheat oven to 350F. *Grease* two loaf pans and set them aside. In a large bowl, *stir together* the flour, baking powder and salt. In another bowl, combine the egg, honey, water and oil. Mix them well. *Peel and chop* the apples into small pieces, but not apple sauce! Add the wet ingredients to the dry, mixing as little as possible. Stir in the apples. Pour into the two loaf pans. *Bake* at 350F for about 40 minutes, until a toothpick comes out dry. When done, remove from the oven. Cool to room temperature, then remove from pans and wrap in aluminum foil. These cakes taste moist and sweet for three days when wrapped in foil. You also can freeze the cakes by putting the foil wrapped cakes in plastic bags and sealing tightly. Defrost in the foil.

Passover Sponge Cake

Milk/Casein Free
Suitable through Stage II

Sponge cake goes with everything. This recipe is easy to make and comes out light and fluffy.   If oranges are a problem, use lemons. Serve with any of the fruit sorbets or sauces.

9 extra large or 10 large to medium eggs

1/2 tsp. sea salt

1 c. unprocessed clover honey

1/2 c. freshly squeezed lemon or orange juice

1/2 c. white matzah meal

1/2 c. whole wheat matzah meal

1/3 c. potato starch

Preheat oven to 325F. *Separate* eggs into two large bowls. Beat the egg whites with an electric mixer at high speed, gradually adding the salt, until the beaten whites form stiff peaks. Set aside. Without cleaning the beaters, *beat* the yolks. *Add* the honey and juice. Beat well. *Combine* in a small bowl the matzah meals and potato starch. Beat the matzah meal/potato starch mixture into the yolk mixture. *Fold* whites into the batter by hand, using care not to beat the air out of the egg whites. Pour into an ungreased tube pan. *Bake* about 1-1/4 hours, until top springs back when touched lightly. Turn pan upside down and cool thoroughly in this position. Carefully remove from pan and place on serving plate.

Pear Cake

Suitable through Stage II

Sweet and rich, this is excellent for company.

4 firm pears

2 c. whole wheat pastry flour

1 tsp. cinnamon

2 T. potato starch

4 T. nonfat, non-instant milk powder

2 tsp. baking powder

1/4 tsp. sea salt

1/2 c. butter

3/4 c. unprocessed clover honey

2 T. freshly squeezed lemon juice, plus enough water to make 3/4 cup

1 egg

Preheat the oven to 350F. *Grease and flour* an 8x8 inch cake pan. *Peel* the pears and slice them into thin slices. Set aside. *Sift* together into a large bowl the flour, cinnamon, potato starch, milk powder, baking powder, and sea salt. In a small bowl, *cream* the butter and the honey. Mix the lemon juice, water and egg into the butter and honey, making sure they are well blended. Mix the wet ingredients into the dry ingredients. *Fold* in the pears. Pour into an 8x8 inch cake pan. Bake at 350F for 30-45 minutes, or until a toothpick comes out dry.

Blueberry Cake

Suitable through Stage II

This is an excellent summer cake for blueberry lovers.

2 c. whole wheat pastry flour

1 tsp. cinnamon

2 T. potato starch

4 T. nonfat, non-instant milk powder

2 tsp. baking powder

1/4 tsp. sea salt

1/2 c. butter

3/4 c. unprocessed clover honey

2 T. freshly squeezed lemon juice, plus enough water to make 3/4 cup

1 egg

2 c. fresh, firm blueberries

Preheat the oven to 350F. *Grease and flour* an 8x8 inch cake pan. *Sift* together into a large bowl the flour, cinnamon, potato starch, milk powder, baking powder, and sea salt. In a small bowl, *cream* the butter and the honey. Mix the lemon juice, water and egg into the butter and honey, making sure they are well blended. Mix the wet ingredients into the dry ingredients. *Fold* in the blueberries. Pour into the cake pan. Bake at 350F for 30-45 minutes, or until a toothpick comes out dry.

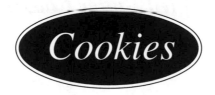

Everyone's Favorite Oatmeal Cookies

Milk/Casein Free
Suitable through Stage II

Finding cookies for kids on restricted diets is hard, but these are terrific. They are great to share with classmates, too. If you do not have time to make the entire batch, you can freeze the cookie dough to use later. The baked cookies also freeze well.

1 c. unsalted butter at room temperature

1-1/2 c. unprocessed clover honey

2 eggs

2-1/2 tsp. baking soda

1 tsp. salt

3 c. whole wheat pastry flour

3 c. old fashioned rolled oats

Preheat the oven to 350F. Put the butter and honey in a bowl. **Beat** them together by hand or with an electric mixer until creamy. Add the remaining ingredients, beating after each one. Drop by teaspoonfuls onto an ungreased cookie sheet. **Bake** at 350F until lightly browned, about 10-12 minutes. Be careful not to overbake the last batch!

Rolled Butter Cookies

Milk/Casein Free (with butter)
Suitable through Stage II

These cookies get rave reviews from kids of all ages. They are great to send to school for parties. Parents and teachers will thank you, because they contain no sugar. This recipe makes 10-13 dozen cookies, depending on how thick the cookies are. **Start these cookies well before you need them. They need to refrigerate before being baked!** If you don't have time to make all the cookies at once, you can freeze the dough to bake later. The baked cookies also freeze well.

> 1-1/2 c. sweet butter at room temperature
>
> 1-1/2 c. unprocessed clover honey
>
> 2 eggs
>
> 1 tsp. baking soda
>
> 4-5 c. whole wheat pastry flour
>
> extra whole wheat pastry flour for kneading

Cream the butter and honey. Mix in the eggs. Add the baking soda and the flour, little by little. Mix well. *Refrigerate* for at least one hour to one day. When you take out the dough, *preheat* the oven to 350F.   Take out a little dough at a time and *knead* some extra flour into it. *Roll out* on a well-floured board or table to about 1/8 inch thickness. *Cut* into desired shapes. If you do not feel like rolling it out, make small balls (about a teaspoonful of dough) and press down with a fork. Or, make a dough log, wrap well in plastic wrap, freeze, then slice off cookies to bake as needed. Whatever method you use, place the cookies on an ungreased cookie sheet. *Bake* at 350F for about 6 minutes until the bottoms are light brown. Do not over bake! Remove immediately to cool.

Valentine's Day Cookies

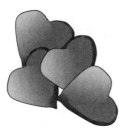

> *Milk/Casein Free (with butter)*
> *Suitable through Stage II*

Looking for something fun for a holiday treat? Try these pink butter cookies. Your kids' friends will love them, as will their teachers—the cookies have no sugar! **Start these cookies well before you need them. They need to refrigerate before being baked!**

1 fresh beet

1/2 c. water

1-1/2 c. sweet butter at room temperature

1-1/2 c. unprocessed clover honey

2 eggs

1 tsp. baking soda

4-5 c. whole wheat pastry flour, plus extra flour for kneading

Peel and cube the beet. Combine it with the 1/2 c. water in a saucepan. Bring to a boil; reduce to simmer and cook until the beet is very soft. Set aside to cool. Puree the beet mixture. In a large bowl, *cream* the butter and honey. Mix in the cool pureed beets and eggs. Add the baking soda and the flour, little by little. Mix well. Add additional flour as needed to stiffen the dough. *Refrigerate* for at least one hour to one day. When you take out the dough, *preheat* the oven to 350F. Take out a little dough at a time and *knead* some extra flour into it. Roll out on a well floured board or table to about 1/8 inch thickness. Cut into heart shapes. Place the cookies on an ungreased cookie sheet. *Bake* at 350F for about 6 minutes until the bottoms are light brown. Do not over bake the last batch! Remove immediately to cool.

Hamantaschen Dough

> *Milk/Casein Free (with butter)*
> *Suitable through Stage II*

"Hamantaschen" are special cookies for the Jewish holiday of Purim, which comes in the late winter. Purim celebrates the victory of the Jewish people over Haman in ancient Persia, who would have had all of the Jews killed. Hamantaschen remind us of "Haman's hat," which, according to accounts, had three corners. The cookies are triangle shaped and filled with delicious fillings, such as *Poppy Seed Filling* or *Pear Sauce* in *Dressings and Sauces*.

These cookies are easy to make, but take a lot of time and patience. The dough must be prepared in advance, and needs to chill for one hour to overnight before filling. This recipe makes 10 to 12 dozen cookies. I prefer to make a very large batch and freeze the cookies for future eating. If a smaller batch is preferred, halve the recipe.

1-3/4 c. unprocessed clover honey

1 c. softened, unsalted butter

2/3 c. expeller pressed safflower oil

6 eggs

2 T. baking powder

1 tsp. salt

10 c. whole wheat pastry flour plus extra for kneading

Cream the honey and butter. Add the oil, then the eggs. Mix well with a wooden spoon. *Mix* the baking powder with some flour and add to the wet mixture. Add the salt. *Mix in the flour* a cup or two at a time, mixing well after each addition. When all the flour is mixed in thoroughly, *refrigerate* at least one hour to overnight. *When ready to use*, preheat the oven to 350F. Break off pieces about the size of two tennis balls. Have sufficient extra flour on hand to knead in extra flour if the dough is too sticky. Roll out one piece at a time to about 1/8 inch thickness. Using a jar lid about 2-1/2 inches in diameter, *cut circles* in the dough. Place about a teaspoonful of filling (*Hamantaschen Poppy Seed Filling* or *Pear Sauce* (found in *Dressings and Sauces*), or make your own from homemade apple sauce or jam) in the center of each circle. You will need one recipe of the *Hamantaschen Poppy Seed Filling*, plus about 3 c. *Pear Sauce*, to fill all the cookies in this recipe. After placing the filling in the center of the circles of dough, *fold up the edges* to form a triangle, pinching the edges of the dough together. Be careful not to get the filling on the edges of the dough or you will not be able to pinch the edges closed. You may need to wet the edges of the dough with a little water to make them stick together. Leave a small opening at the top so you can see the filling. *Bake* at 350F for about 10 minutes, or until the edges and bottoms are slightly brown.

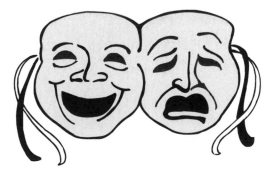

Hamantaschen Poppy Seed Filling

> *Wheat/Gluten Free*
> *Milk/Casein Free (with butter)*
> *Egg Free*
> *Suitable through Stage III*

"Hamantaschen" are special filled cookies for the Jewish holiday of Purim. This is a recipe for traditional poppy seed (mohn) filling, and makes enough filling for about 6-8 dozen cookies made from *Hamantaschen Dough*. Poppy seeds are available in bulk from health food stores and cooperatives.

   3 c. poppy seeds

   2 c. water

   2 T. butter

   1 c. unprocessed clover honey

Place the poppy seeds, water and butter in a 3 quart saucepan. Heat on medium until the water boils. Simmer until water is absorbed. Add the honey. Continue heating, and mixing every once in awhile, until most of the liquid from the honey is absorbed. Cool, then fill *Hamantaschen Dough*. Enjoy!

Scandinavian Whole Wheat Butter Cookies

Milk/Casein Free (with butter)
Suitable through Stage II

These are butter cookies with a difference. They are sweet, but not too sweet, and have a texture that is both light and rich. Makes 6-7 dozen cookies.

  1 c. sweet butter

  1 c. unprocessed clover honey

  1 egg

  1-1/2 c. whole wheat pastry flour

  1-1/2 c. potato starch flour ("kartoffel mel")

Preheat the oven to 375F. *Cream* the butter and honey. Mix in the egg. *Sift* the flour and potato starch flour. Mix the dry mixture into the wet mixture. *Refrigerate* mixture at least one hour. *Drop* by teaspoonfuls onto an ungreased cookie sheet, making sure the cookies are 2 inches apart. They spread during baking! Bake at 375F for approximately 9 minutes, or until edges begin to brown. Remove from cookie sheet to cool.

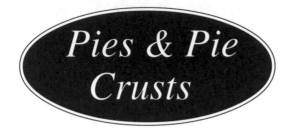

Whole Wheat Oil Pie Crust

> *Cholesterol Free*
> *Milk/Casein Free*
> *Egg Free*
> *Suitable through Stage II*

This is a basic pie crust for a nine inch single crust pie. I use oil for those who do not like or cannot have a butter crust. It is very crumbly and is pressed into the pan rather than rolled out. This recipe makes enough crust for a shallow 9 inch pie. For a deep dish 10 inch pie, double the recipe.

1-1/4 c. whole wheat pastry flour

1/2 tsp. salt

1/3 c. expeller pressed safflower oil

3-6 T. freezing cold water

Mix the flour with the salt, then thoroughly mix in the oil. The mixture will be very wet, but don't worry. Do not think that you shouldn't add water! The water binds the oil and flour together. After mixing in the oil, *add* water one tablespoonful at a time. *Mix* until crust is the consistency of gooey clay and holds together. *Press* into a 9" pie plate. Increase the recipe proportionately for larger pie shells. Fill and bake according to instructions in your pie recipe.

Whole Wheat Butter Pie Crust

Milk/Casein Free (with butter)
Egg Free
Suitable through Stage II

This butter pie crust recipe makes one nine inch pie. Although the crust is heavier than the oil crust, it is tasty and disappears every time it's served!

1/2 tsp. sea salt

1-1/4 c. whole wheat pastry flour

3/4 c. sweet cream butter, cold

3-6 T. freezing cold water

Mix flour and salt. *Cut* in the butter with a pastry blender, until the mixture balls up the size of peas. *Add* water one tablespoonful at a time. Mix until mixture forms a ball. *Roll out* or press into a 9" pie plate. Increase the recipe for large pie shells. Fill and bake according to directions in your pie recipe.

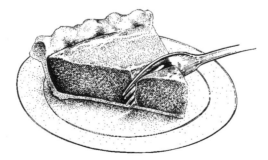

Spicy Non-Dairy Pumpkin Pie Filling

Wheat/Gluten Free
Milk/Casein Free
Suitable through Stage IV

Your Thanksgiving guests will love this superb dairy free pie. Bake one day in advance and let the flavor settle in. Makes enough filling for one 9-inch pie crust. For a deep dish, 10-inch pie crust, double the recipe. You might end up with a small amount left over, which you can bake in some muffin tins for "pie-ettes."

   3/4 c. unprocessed clover honey

   1/2 tsp. salt

   1/2 tsp. cinnamon

   1/8 to 1/2 tsp. mace

   1/2 tsp. powdered ginger or 1/4 tsp. fresh chopped ginger

   1/4 tsp. powdered cloves

   2 eggs

   2 T. melted butter (optional)

   1-1/2 c. cooked, pureed pie pumpkin

   9" pie unbaked pie crust, using your favorite recipe from this cookbook

Preheat the oven to 425F. **Prepare the pumpkin** according to directions in **A Note on Ingredients**. **Mix** all ingredients (except the pastry shell) with an electric mixer. When mixing in the spices, keep in mind that the mace makes the pie very spicy. For milder pies, put in 1/8 tsp. mace. For very spicy pies, put in 1/2 tsp. mace. For pies in between, put in varying amounts to suit your taste. **Pour** into the pastry shell. To protect edges of shell from burning, cover the edges with aluminum foil tents. Bake 15 minutes at 425F, then reduce heat to 350F and bake another 40 minutes, or until toothpick comes out dry. Cool before eating.

Rice Pie Crust with Oil

Cholesterol Free
Wheat/Gluten Free
Milk/Casein Free
Egg Free
Suitable through Stage IV

This is a tasty crust for a double crusted 9- or 10-inch pie.

3 c. Ener-G Rice Mix or brown rice flour

1/2 tsp. sea salt

2/3 c. expeller pressed safflower oil

up to 1-1/2 c. ice water

Mix rice mix and salt in a large bowl. *Add* the oil and mix thoroughly so the rice mix/oil mixture resembles small pebbles. *Add the water*, a little at a time, and stir. Add just enough water to get a consistency like clay, where you can press the dough into a pie pan and have it hold together. Usually about 1 c. of ice water is sufficient, but this depends on the humidity in the house. *Press* half of the dough into a 9 or 10 inch pie pan for the bottom crust. *Fill* the crust with your favorite pie filling. *Press* the remaining crust into small pieces and lay across the top of the filling, or crumble the remaining crust over the top. Follow baking directions for your pie filling, or *bake* at 350F for about an hour. The pie is done when fruit filling bubbles through cracks in the crust.

Thanksgiving Pie

> *Milk/Casein Free*
> *Suitable through Stage II*

A beautiful addition to the Thanksgiving table, light and delicious.

Pastry (for top and bottom crusts)

2-1/4 c. whole wheat pastry flour

1 c. sweet butter

1 egg yolk

2 T. fresh lemon juice (not bottled!)

1/2 c. water

1 egg white plus 1 T. of water

Preheat the oven to 400F. Make the pastry: Cut the butter into the flour until the mixture forms pea-sized balls. Set aside. *Beat* the egg yolk with the lemon juice and water. *Mix* the wet ingredients into the flour until it is a doughy consistency. The dough will be very wet and sticky. You may be tempted to add extra flour. DON'T DO IT!! *Set the pastry aside* and continue with filling.

Filling:

4 firm pears

1 c. fresh, whole cranberries

1/4 c. whole wheat pastry flour

1 tsp. cinnamon

3/4 c. unprocessed clover honey

To make the filling: First, peel and slice the pears into very thin slices. Mix in the remaining filling ingredients. Then, ***press half of the pastry*** into a 9 inch Pyrex pie pan or a 7x11 inch Pyrex baking dish. ***Fill*** with filling. ***Beat the egg white*** with the water. Pour over fruit. ***Press*** pieces of the top pastry between your fingers and lay them over the fruit, covering the fruit as best you can. ***Bake*** at 400F for 50 minutes.

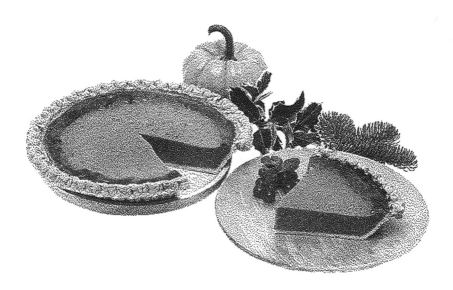

Fruit Pie

*Milk/Casein Free
Suitable through Stage II*

This is a variation on an old favorite. You can make it using any fresh, not overly ripe summer fruit.

Pastry (for top and bottom crusts):

2-1/4 c. whole wheat pastry flour

1 c. sweet (unsalted) cold butter

1 egg, separated

2 T. freshly squeezed lemon juice

1/2 c. water

1 T. water

Preheat the oven to 400F. *Make the pastry:* Cut the butter into the flour until the mixture forms pea-sized balls. Set aside. Beat the egg yolk with the lemon juice and water. Mix this wet mixture into the flour until it is a doughy consistency. The dough will be very wet and sticky. You might be tempted to add extra flour. DON'T DO IT!! *Set aside and make the filling.*

Continued on facing page. . . . .

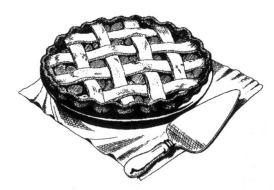

Filling:

5 c. fresh or freshly frozen whole berries, or peeled and sliced fresh fruit

1/4 c. whole wheat pastry flour

1 tsp. cinnamon

3/4 c. unprocessed clover honey

Mix all of the filling ingredients together. *Divide* the pastry in half. *Press* half of the pastry into a 9 inch Pyrex pie pan or a 7x11 inch Pyrex dish. *Fill* with filling. Beat the egg white with the water. *Pour* over the filling. *Press* pieces of the second half of the pastry dough between your fingers and lay them over the fruit, overlapping the pieces to cover the fruit. Bake at 400F for 50 minutes. The fruit should be bubbling.

Blueberry Pie Filling For Double Crusted Pie

Cholesterol Free
Wheat/Gluten Free
Milk/Casein Free
Egg Free
Suitable through Stage IV

5 c. fresh or freshly frozen blueberries

3/4 c. unprocessed clover honey

1/4 c. brown rice flour

Defrost frozen blueberries. Mix all ingredients together. Fill an unbaked 9 inch pie crust. Layer a top crust, making sure there are openings in the crust. Bake at 350F to 375F for 60 minutes, until the berries are bubbling through the crust and the crust is light brown.

Pears 'N Honey Matzah Pie

Milk/Casein Free
Egg Free
Suitable through Stage II

This pie is tasty on the Jewish holiday of Passover, when conventional baked goods are limited, but can be eaten all year round.

Crust:

5 whole wheat matzah boards

1/2 c. (1 stick) unsalted butter

1/4 tsp. cinnamon

5 T. unprocessed clover honey

water

Preheat the oven to 350F. Make the crust first. In a medium sized bowl, **break** the matzah into small pieces. **Cover** them with water and let them soak a few minutes until they are soft. Meanwhile, **melt the butter** in a saucepan. **Drain** the matzah well by squeezing the water out. **Mix** in the butter and honey. If the mixture is too dry, add water. Mix in the cinnamon. Set aside. Now make the filling.

Filling:

5 firm pears

2 T. unprocessed clover honey

1/4 tsp. cinnamon

Peel and slice the pears. Mix with the honey, butter and cinnamon mixture. Use a ten-inch Pyrex pie pan. *Spread* half of the matzah mixture on the bottom of the pan. *Fill* with the pear mixture. Then *spread* on the remaining matzah mixture. Cover with aluminum foil. *Bake* at 350F for about 40 min. to an hour, or until the pears are very bubbly and soft. The pie should steam when the foil is removed.

Baked Crustless Blueberry Pie

Cholesterol Free
Wheat/Gluten Free
Milk/Casein Free
Egg Free
Suitable through Stage IV

Do you know people who only eat the pie filling and leave the crust? This pie is for them!

  4-5 c. blueberries, fresh or freshly frozen

  1/2c. - 3/4 c. unprocessed clover honey

  1/4 c. Mochi white rice flour

Preheat the oven to 350F. *Combine* all ingredients in an oven safe bowl or souffle dish. Use less honey for a less sweet dessert, and more honey for a sweeter dessert. *Cover* tightly with aluminum foil. *Bake* at 350F until the pie is bubbling, about an hour for fresh blueberries, longer for frozen.

Instant Crustless Blueberry Pie for One

> *Cholesterol Free*
> *Wheat/Gluten Free*
> *Milk/Casein Free*
> *Egg Free*
> *Suitable through Stage IV*

This recipe makes a small amount of crustless pie for people who just love pie filling and can't wait to eat it. It's quick and easy, taking about 6 minutes to make. This is a great kid recipe.

   1 c. fresh or freshly frozen blueberries

   1/4 c. unprocessed clover honey

   1 T. Mochi white rice flour

Mix the blueberries and honey in a microwaveable bowl that has enough room to boil without splattering. *Microwave* on high for one minute. *Stir.* *Add* the rice flour little by little, mixing well after each addition. *Microwave* for two minutes on high. *Stir.* *Microwave* for one minute on high. Cool to a comfortable temperature, then gobble up.

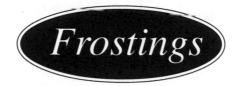

Honey Butter Cream Frosting

Egg Free
Suitable through Stage II

This is an exceptionally good frosting, even though it uses no flavorings other than honey and butter. If dairy is unacceptable, you can use water.

> *either*: 1 c. water *plus* 1/4 c. nonfat, non-instant dry milk powder *or* 1 c. milk
>
> 1/4 c. unsifted, unbleached white flour
>
> 1 c. butter at room temperature
>
> 1 c. unprocessed clover honey
>
> 1 tsp. freshly squeezed lemon juice

If using dry milk: Combine dry milk and flour in saucepan. Mix well. Add 1 c. water. Whisk. *If using regular milk*: Combine milk and flour in saucepan. Whisk. *Continue for all ingredients*: *Heat* over medium heat, stirring constantly, until the mixture boils and thickens. Remove. *Cool* to room temperature. In a separate bowl, *cream* the butter and honey until fluffy. Be sure the flour and milk have cooled completely before combining the butter/honey with the flour/milk , or the butter will melt. *Add* the butter/honey to the flour/milk, beating with an electric mixer at medium speed until frosting is very fluffy. *Beat* in the lemon juice. *Spread* over a cool cake. Refrigerate until ready to serve.

Fun and Flavorful Butter Cream Frosting

Egg Free
Suitable through Stage II

Need a treat for your kids, but food coloring is a problem? Never fear. They'll love this frosting. You can make fun colors that taste great. Consider the possibilities of other brightly colored fruits and vegetables.   Just follow the same directions, substituting your fruit or vegetable of choice. Keep in mind that both tomatoes and beets are sweet. You will need to increase the honey if using other vegetables.

For orange frosting:

1 tomato

water

1/4 c. unsifted, unbleached white flour

1 c. butter at room temperature

1 c. unprocessed clover honey

For pink frosting:

1 beet

water

1/4 c. unsifted, unbleached white flour

1 c. butter at room temperature

1 c. unprocessed clover honey

Prepare the beet or tomato: Peel, if necessary, cut, and place in a small saucepan with enough water to prevent burning, and cooking until very soft. *Puree* in a blender. Combine the pureed mixture with white flour in saucepan. *Heat* over medium heat, stirring constantly, until it boils and thickens. Remove. *Cool* to

room temperature. While the flour mixture is cooling, **cream** the
butter and honey in another bowl, until fluffy. Before adding to
the flour mixture, be sure the flour and milk have cooled
completely, or the butter will melt. ***Add*** the butter/honey to the
flour/milk, beating at medium speed until frosting is very fluffy.
Spread over cake or cookies that have cooled completely, or the
frosting will melt. Refrigerate until serving.

Honey Butter Frosting

Wheat/Gluten Free
Milk/Casein Free
Egg Free
Suitable through Stage IV

Birthdays call for frosting. This one is easy to make, tastes great
and looks especially great even on top of ***Sorbet Birthday Cake***.
Because the frosting is so sweet, use it sparingly by placing it
judiciously around the edges of the cake or sorbet and using the
frosting for writing on a dark background.

- 1 c. unprocessed clover honey

- 1 c. sweet, unsalted butter at room temperature

- 2 T. freshly squeezed lemon juice

With an electric mixer, cream the butter, lemon juice and the
honey thoroughly. Put into a cake decorator and frost the edges of
your cake or sorbet cake. Use a large syringe to write with the
frosting. Refrigerate or refreeze immediately.

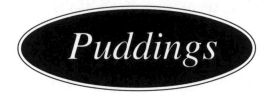

Creamy Pudding

Wheat/Gluten Free
Suitable through Stage II

Our family loves pudding.   This one is sweet and simple, but very creamy and delicious. The pudding takes only about 12 minutes to make, despite the lengthy directions. Do not double.

   2 egg yolks

   1/2 c. nonfat, non-instant dry milk powder

   3-1/2 T. potato starch

   2 c. water

   2-4 T. unprocessed clover honey

   2 T. butter (optional)

   1/8 tsp. cinnamon (optional)

Lightly beat the egg yolks in a medium glass bowl. Set aside but within an arm's reach. In a 2 quart saucepan, thoroughly ***mix*** the milk powder and potato starch. ***Add*** 1/4 c. of the water, mixing well, preferably with a whisk. Both the potato starch and the milk powder have a tendency to form lumps. *Add* remaining water 1/4 c. at a time, mixing after each addition. After adding all the water, turn the heat to medium and begin stirring. *Stir continuously* while the mixture heats to a boil. Do not hurry the process by turning heat up higher, as the mixture will burn. Almost all at once, the mixture will thicken. *Continue* cooking until it boils. Remove from heat.

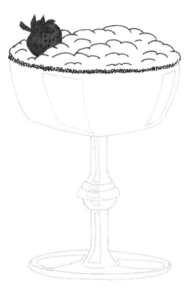

Gradually mix a little of the saucepan mixture to the egg yolks in the glass bowl. Then, put the saucepan back on the heat. *Pour* the egg mixture back into the saucepan. Mix thoroughly. *While stirring constantly*, heat to boiling. *Pour* the mixture back into the glass bowl. *Add* cinnamon and butter, if desired, stirring the butter until it melts. Stir well. When the pudding has cooled off a little, *stir* in the honey one tablespoonful at a time. Stir in just enough to barely sweeten the pudding, as too much honey will cause the pudding to become watery. The pudding is now ready. Serve as soon as the pudding is cool enough to eat.

Blueberry Flummery

> *Cholesterol Free*
> *Wheat/Gluten Free*
> *Milk/Casein Free*
> *Egg Free*
> *Suitable through Stage IV*

Flummery is a thick, creamy fruit pudding, made without dairy or eggs. It was a popular dessert in the 1700s, and can be made with any type of berry. Use this recipe as a guide for other types of berries.

2 c. blueberries

3/4 c. water

1/2 c. + 2 T. unprocessed clover honey

4 T. sweet Mochi rice thickener

8 T. hot water

Place the blueberries, water and honey in a 2-quart saucepan. Slowly bring to a boil, then reduce to a simmer. Cook for 10 minutes. While the berries are cooking, *mix* the Mochi rice thickener with the hot water, a few teaspoonfuls at a time, mixing while adding the water. You will have a thick, gooey paste. When the berries are cooked, reduce the heat. *Slowly drizzle* in the rice paste, stirring or whisking the berry mixture constantly. Do not let the rice paste clump up. When you have added all the rice paste, continue stirring for another minute. Continue cooking on low heat for 10 minutes, stirring occasionally. Pour into custard cups and cool for at least 20 minutes before serving. The flummery thickens as it cools. Makes approximately four half-cup servings. Serve warm or cold.

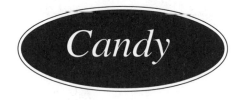

Caramel

> *Wheat/Gluten Free*
> *Milk/Casein Free (with butter)*
> *Egg Free*
> *Suitable through Stage IV*

This plain caramel is delicious and sticky sweet.

> 1 c. sweet butter
> 1 c. unprocessed clover honey

Place the butter and honey together in a saucepan. ***Heat*** over medium heat, stirring constantly. Let the mixture come to a rolling boil, being careful not to burn. The mixture will caramelize in about 10 minutes. Cook until a few drops hold their shape when dropped into cold water. ***Remove*** from heat. ***Remove*** from pan with a greased rubber spatula and pour onto plastic wrap on a cookie sheet. ***Cool*** to room temperature. Do not cool in the freezer. When cool, cut into smaller pieces and wrap in plastic wrap for individual candies.

Honey Crunch Candy

> *Milk/Casein Free*
> *Egg Free*
> *Wheat/Gluten Free (with alterations)*
> *Suitable through Stage IV*

Kids and adults both love to crunch on this candy. This is a great treat to send to school for those sugar laden celebrations.

1 c. unprocessed clover honey

1/2 c. sweet butter

2 c. "Nature-O's" by Arrowhead Mills or similar sugar free oat cereal (if on Stage III or IV, substitute Puffed Rice for all cereal)

1/2 c. whole grain Puffed Wheat or Puffed Rice cereal

optional: 1/2 c. rolled oats (for Stages I and II)

extra butter, expeller pressed safflower oil or cooking spray for greasing

Put the honey and the butter in a 2-quart saucepan. Turn on medium heat. Stirring constantly, bring the mixture to a rolling boil. Keep stirring at a rolling boil for 7-12 minutes, until the mixture caramelizes. It will become very gooey and change color. *Remove* from heat. *Mix* in the cereal. The "Nature-O's" provide crunch; the puffed wheat or rice provide good texture— they add air. *Grease*, with butter, oil, or oil-spray, an 8x8 inch pan or pie pan. With a greased rubber spatula, press the mixture into the pan. Cool slowly (do not freeze). When cool, cut the candy into small squares, not larger than 2x2 inches. If you are not eating the candy immediately, wrap each piece in a small piece of plastic. Put all the pieces in a plastic bag and refrigerate or freeze until you are ready to use them. These candies are super sweet, and super tasty.

*The "Nature-O's" are very crunchy and good, and are unsweetened. As of the date we wrote this book, this cereal is the only packaged cereal of this type that contains no offending sweeteners, such as sugar, concentrated fruit juice, or barley malt.

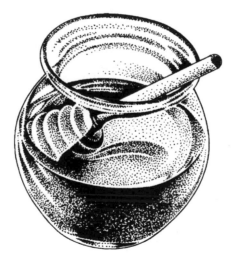

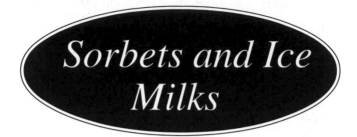

Raspberry Sorbet

> *Cholesterol Free*
> *Wheat/Gluten Free*
> *Milk/Casein Free*
> *Egg Free*
> *Suitable through Stage IV*

Red raspberry sorbet is sweet and light, and a beautiful deep pink color. You need a food blender or processor to start the sorbet and an ice-cream maker to complete the processing. Use fresh or freshly frozen fruit (see *A Note on Ingredients*).

2 c. fresh or freshly frozen raspberries

1 c. unprocessed clover honey

1 c. water

Put the berries, honey and water in the blender or food processor. For a blender, start at the lowest speed, then after a few seconds move the speed to the highest. For a food processor, process at high speed. *Process until the mixture is smooth* and you cannot see any chunks of berry skin. *Pour* the mixture into the ice-cream part of your ice cream maker. *Process* according to directions for ice cream. The mixture will be the consistency of soft serve ice cream, but will harden after freezing. Serve immediately, or transfer to another container.

Triple Berry Sorbet

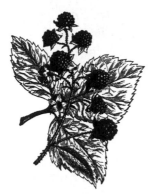

Cholesterol Free
Wheat/Gluten Free
Milk/Casein Free
Egg Free
Suitable through Stage IV

The flavor of this sorbet is simply divine. Sorbet is a great alternative to traditional ice cream. It is acceptable on even the most limited food regimens. You need a food blender or processor to start the sorbet and an ice-cream maker to complete the processing. Use fresh or fresh frozen fruit (see *A Note on Ingredients*).

 1 c. fresh or freshly frozen raspberries

 1 c. fresh or freshly frozen sweet blackberries

 1 pint fresh or freshly frozen blueberries

 1 c. unprocessed clover honey

 1 c. water

Put the berries, honey and water in the blender or food processor. For a blender, start at the lowest speed, then after a few seconds move the speed to the highest. For a food processor, process at high speed. *Process* for several minutes until the mixture is smooth and you cannot see any chunks of berry skin. *Pour* the mixture into the ice cream part of your ice-cream maker. Process according to directions for ice cream. The mixture will be like soft-serve ice cream, which will harden when frozen. Serve immediately or transfer to another container and freeze.

Blueberry Sorbet

> *Cholesterol Free*
> *Wheat/Gluten Free*
> *Milk/Casein Free*
> *Egg Free*
> *Suitable through Stage IV*

Summer is a wonderful time for frozen treats. We serve this sorbet to our children's friends all of the time. You need a food blender or processor to start the sorbet and an ice-cream maker to complete the processing. Use fresh or fresh frozen fruit (see *A Note on Ingredients*). Makes about 1-1/2 quarts.

4 c. fresh or freshly frozen blueberries (in season)

1 c. unprocessed clover honey

2 c. water, divided in half

Put the blueberries, honey and 1 c. water in the blender or food processor. For a blender, start at the lowest speed, then after a few seconds move the speed to the highest. For a food processor, process at high speed. *Process* for several minutes, until the mixture is smooth and you cannot see any chunks of blueberry skin. *Pour* the mixture into the ice-cream part of your ice-cream maker. Add the additional water only if the mixture looks too thick. You may need to experiment to determine the proper amount of water for your ice-cream maker. *Process* according to your ice cream maker's directions for ice cream. The mixture will make soft serve type sorbet which will harden after frozen. Serve immediately or transfer to another container and freeze.

Cantaloupe Sorbet

Cholesterol Free
Wheat/Gluten Free
Milk/Casein Free
Egg Free
Suitable through Stage III

Not really! If you love cantaloupe, you will love this sorbet even more. The sorbet comes out a lovely light orange color, which works well in the *Sorbet Birthday Cake.* You need both a blender or food processor and an ice cream maker to make this recipe. Makes about 1 quart of sorbet:

> 1/2 large, or 1 small cantaloupe
>
> 1/2 c. unprocessed clover honey
>
> 1 c. water

Peel, seed and chop the cantaloupe into large chunks. *Put the fruit,* honey and water in the blender or food processor. For a blender, start at the lowest speed, then after a few seconds move the speed to the highest. For a food processor, process at high speed. *Process* until the mixture is smooth. *Pour* the mixture into the ice-cream part of your ice-cream maker. *Process* according to directions for ice cream. The mixture will be the consistency of soft serve ice cream, but will harden after freezing. Serve immediately, or transfer to another container and freeze.

Blueberry Pear Sorbet

Cholesterol Free
Wheat/Gluten Free
Milk/Casein Free
Egg Free
Suitable through Stage III

This is lighter and slightly sweeter than plain blueberry sorbet, but like blueberry sorbet, it is delicious and wonderful to eat for everyone. You need both a food processor or blender and an ice cream maker to complete this recipe. Use only fresh or freshly frozen berries (see *A Note on Ingredients*). This recipe makes about 1-1/2 quarts of sorbet.

2 firm pears, peeled, cored and chopped

2 c. fresh or fresh frozen blueberries

1/2 c. unprocessed clover honey

1 c. water

Combine all ingredients in a blender or food processor, and process on high until the mixture is smooth and totally liquefied. *Pour* mixture into the ice cream cylinder of your ice cream maker and *process* according to directions. The mixture will be the consistency of soft serve ice cream, but will harden after freezing. Serve immediately, or transfer to another container and freeze.

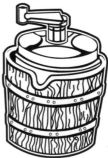

Blueberry Orange Sorbet

> *Cholesterol Free*
> *Wheat/Gluten Free*
> *Milk/Casein Free*
> *Egg Free*
> *Suitable through Stage III*

Sweet and tangy describes this unusual sorbet. Makes about 2 quarts of sorbet.

  4 c. fresh or freshly frozen blueberries

  1/2 c. freshly squeezed orange juice

  1/2 c. unprocessed clover honey

  1-2 c. water

Combine fruit, juice, honey and one cup of water in a blender or food processor, and process on high until the mixture is smooth and totally liquefied. *Pour* the mixture into the ice cream cylinder of your ice cream maker. *If the mixture* looks very thick, add 1 c. water. The amount of water you need varies with the type of ice cream maker you have. You may need to experiment. *Process* according to directions. The mixture will be the consistency of soft serve ice cream, but will harden after freezing. Serve immediately, or transfer to another container and freeze.

Mandarin Pear Sorbet

> *Cholesterol Free*
> *Wheat/Gluten Free*
> *Milk/Casein Free*
> *Egg Free*
> *Suitable through Stage III*

This is a surprising winter dessert, when pears and tangerines are in season. This is especially tasty with Clementine mandarin oranges.

> 5 firm Bartlett or D'Anjou pears
>
> 2 seedless tangerines or mandarin oranges
>
> 1/2 c. water
>
> 1/2 c. unprocessed clover honey

Peel and chop the pears. Peel the oranges and break into sections. *Combine* all ingredients in a blender. *Blend* on high for a few minutes, until thoroughly liquefied and no chunks of fruit are apparent. *Pour* into an ice-cream maker and process as directed. The mixture will be the consistency of soft serve ice cream, but will harden after freezing. Serve immediately, or transfer to another container and freeze. Makes about 1-1/2 quarts.

Blueberry Popsicles

> *Cholesterol Free*
> *Wheat/Gluten Free*
> *Milk/Casein Free*
> *Egg Free*
> *Suitable through Stage IV*

 1 pint blueberries

 1/2 c. water

 1/2 c. unprocessed clover honey

Blend all ingredients in a blender on high. Pour into popsicle molds to the line on the molds. Freeze. Makes eight 2-oz. popsicles.

Freshly Frozen Berries

> *Cholesterol Free*
> *Wheat/Gluten Free*
> *Milk/Casein Free*
> *Egg Free*
> *Suitable through Stage IV*

Many of the desserts in this book depend on fresh fruit. You can freeze berries during the summer so they are available all year.

 Fresh blueberries, raspberries, and/or blackberries, any
 quantity (Stages I and II may also use strawberries)

Sort the berries to eliminate any moldy ones. Unless you are confident that the berries are clean, wash and drip dry. The berries must be dry before freezing. Place on a cookie sheet or other pan that fits in your freezer. Make sure the berries don't touch each other. Place the cookie sheet in the freezer. When the berries are frozen, put them in plastic bags, seal, and store in freezer until you are ready to use them.

Birthday Sorbet Cake

> *Cholesterol Free*
> *Wheat/Gluten Free*
> *Milk/Casein Free*
> *Egg Free*
> *Suitable through Stages III-IV*

Birthday cakes are hard to find when you need something without wheat, dairy and eggs! We use different colored sorbets to create patterns in a pan. Decorate with *Honey Butter Frosting*.

One recipe of each, two different colors of sorbet, paying careful attention to their suitability for your stages. For example:

> *Cantaloupe Sorbet* and *Blueberry Sorbet*
>
> *Raspberry Sorbet* and *Blueberry Sorbet*
>
> *Cantaloupe Sorbet* and *Triple Berry Sorbet*

For Checkerboard: Allow the first color of sorbet to soften, but not melt. Place squares of the sorbet into a 9x13 inch pan in a checkerboard pattern, with the second color missing. Freeze for a few hours. Then soften, but do not melt, the second color of sorbet and fill in the missing spaces on your checkerboard. Freeze until just before serving. *For A Rainbow Pattern*: Soften the first color of sorbet, spread half of it in the pan, refreeze; then repeat with the second color, layering it over the first color, repeating with different colors until the pan is full. The top layer will be a uniform color, but when you cut the dessert, you will have a beautiful rainbow. *If frosting*, choose an appropriate frosting. Squeeze the frosting through a decorator tube to accent the cake. Refreeze until you are ready to serve.

Blueberry Ice Milk

> *Cholesterol Free*
> *Wheat/Gluten Free*
> *Egg Free*
> *Suitable through Stage II*

This is a rich, fruity ice milk, which derives its sweetness from the fruit and milk.

3 firm pears

2 c. firm blueberries

1 c. nonfat milk

1-1/2 c. non-instant, nonfat milk powder

Peel, core and chop the pears. Place them with the berries and liquid milk in a blender or food processor and *process* on high until all ingredients are totally smooth. *Add the milk powder* a little at a time, processing after each addition. Make sure you do not add the milk powder all at once, or it turns into a cement-like

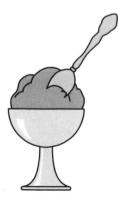

substance that is extremely difficult to work with. *Process* until the entire mixture is smooth. *Pour* mixture into the ice cream cylinder of your ice cream maker, and process according to directions. The mixture will be the consistency of soft serve ice cream, but will harden after freezing. Serve immediately, or transfer to another container and freeze.

Cherry Ice Milk

> *Cholesterol Free*
> *Wheat/Gluten Free*
> *Egg Free*
> *Suitable through Stage II*

Cherries and milk, the essence of summer, in a tempting combination!

- 3 firm pears
- 2 c. ripe, pitted cherries
- 1 c. nonfat milk
- 1-1/2 c. non-instant, nonfat milk powder

Peel, core and chop the pears. Place them with the cherries and liquid milk in a blender or food processor and *process* on high until all ingredients are smooth and liquefied. *Add the milk powder* a little at a time, processing after each addition. Make sure you do not add the milk powder all at once, or it turns into a cement-like substance that is extremely difficult to work with. *Process* until the entire mixture is smooth. *Pour* mixture into the ice cream cylinder of your ice cream maker, and process according to directions. The mixture will be the consistency of soft serve ice cream, but will harden after freezing. Serve immediately, or transfer to another container and freeze.

Spicy Pear Ice Milk

Cholesterol Free
Wheat/Gluten Free
Egg Free
Suitable through Stage II

Enjoy the taste of ice-cream without the sugar and fat. This recipe can be made fresh all year.

6 firm pears

either 1-1/2 c. non-instant, nonfat milk powder plus 1 c. water *or* 2 c. milk

3/4 tsp. cinnamon

Peel, core and chop the pears into chunks. Put them in a blender or food processor and begin processing on high. When the pears are pureed, *start mixing in* the milk powder and the water, alternately, processing after each addition. If you add the milk powder too quickly, it turns into a cement like substance that is extremely difficult to work with. *If you are using milk* instead of milk powder, pour in the milk. *Add* the cinnamon. *Process* until the entire mixture is smooth. *Pour* mixture into the ice cream cylinder of your ice cream maker, and process according to directions. The mixture will be the consistency of soft serve ice cream, but will harden after freezing. Serve immediately, or transfer to another container and freeze.

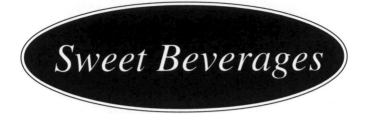

Sweet Beverages

Hot Spicy Milk

Wheat/Gluten Free
Egg Free
Suitable through Stage II

This is a great drink in the winter, created by a our daughter seeking an alternative to hot chocolate.

1 c. milk

(regular milk if tolerable; otherwise, use 1 c. hot water plus 4 T. nonfat, non-instant dry milk, mixed well)

1/16 tsp. cinnamon

1/16 tsp. allspice

1/16 tsp. cloves

Combine all ingredients in a mug. Heat in microwave on high for 1 minute, 15 seconds. Stir. Serve immediately.

Fresh Cold Lemonade

> *Cholesterol Free*
> *Wheat/Gluten Free*
> *Milk/Casein Free*
> *Egg Free*
> *Suitable through Stage IV*

Picnics, holidays, parties, or just fun times demand special drinks. For those who love lemonade, this recipe is sure to be a favorite. Although this recipe makes a gallon, you can decrease it proportionately to the size of your container.

    2 c. freshly squeezed lemon juice

    2 c. unprocessed clover honey

    4 c. boiling water

    additional water

In a one gallon jar, mix the lemon juice, honey and 4 c. boiling water. When the honey is completely dissolved, add enough additional water to fill the jar. Refrigerate until very cold, then serve.

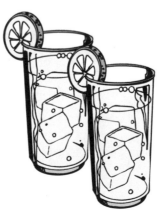

Hot Lemonade

Cholesterol Free
Wheat/Gluten Free
Milk/Casein Free
Egg Free
Suitable through Stage IV

Nothing hits the spot like hot lemonade on a cold day. For teatime or anytime.

boiling water

2 tsp. freshly squeezed lemon juice

1 tsp. unprocessed clover honey

Put the lemon juice in a mug. Add boiling water to fill the mug to a comfortable level. Mix in the honey. Enjoy!

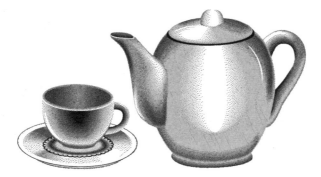

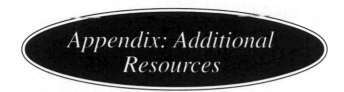

Appendix: Additional Resources

Suggestions for Further Reading:

Sidney Baker, M.D., *Detoxification and Healing* (New Canaan, Conn.: Keats Publishing, Inc.), c. 1997; see also *Notes on the Yeast Problem* (no longer in print).

Dr. James F. Balch, and Phyllis A. Balch, *Prescription for Nutritional Healing* (Garden City, New York: Avery Publishing Group), c. 1997.

Mary Callahan, *Fighting for Tony*

William Crook, M.D., *The Yeast Connection Handbook: How Yeasts Can Make You Feel Sick All Over and the Steps You Need to Take to Regain Your Health* (Jackson, TN: Professional Books, Inc.), c. 1997, 1998, 1999.

William Crook, M.D., *The Yeast Connection and the Woman* (Jackson, TN: Professional Books, Inc.), c.1995.

Udo Erasmus, *Fats that Heal, Fats that Kill: The Complete Guide to Fats, Oils, Cholesterol and Human Health* (Alive Books), 1998.

Ann Louise Gittleman, *Beyond Pritikin: A Total Nutrition Program for Rapid Weight Loss, Longevity and Good Health* (Bantam Books), 1996.

William Shaw, Ph.D, *Biological Treatments for Autism and PDD: What's going on? What can you do about it?*, with contributions from Bruce Semon, M.D., Ph.D., Lisa Lewis, Ph.D., Karyn Seroussi and Pamela Scott, (Great Plains Laboratory) 1998. (This book is available through the Wisconsin Institute of Nutrition, www. nutritioninstitute.com.)

C. Orian Truss, *The Missing Diagnosis*, c. 1982, available from the author, P.O. Box 26508, Birmingham, Alabama 35226

Testing for Yeast and Allergies:

The Great Plains Laboratory
9335 W. 75th Street
Overland Park, KS 66204
(913) 341-8949
www.greatplainslaboratory.com

Resources on Autism and other Medical Conditions:

There are many resources on autism. We recommend starting
with the most comprehensive clearinghouse for, and source of
information on, autism. Autism Research Institute publishes a
quarterly newsletter, available for a nominal subscription fee. Its
website has links to most of the major sources of information
regarding autism.

Autism Research Institute
4182 Adams Avenue
San Diego, CA 92116
www.autism.com/ari

The website of Wisconsin Institute of Nutrition, publisher of
Feast Without Yeast, also has information about autism, as well as
many other medical conditions mentioned in this book, including
Attention Deficit Disorder, Multiple Sclerosis, Eczema,
Rheumatoid Arthritis, and other conditions. See
www.nutritioninstitute.com.

Specialized Food Products:

If unavailable through your local health food store or food cooperative, contact the company to find out who distributes these
products in your area.

Pastariso brand rice pasta: Rice Innovations, Inc., 1773 Bayly
Street, Pickering, Ontario, Canada, L1W 2Y7

Ener-G Foods: Ener-G Foods, P.O. Box 84487, Seattle, WA
98124-5787

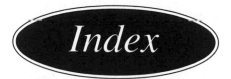
Index

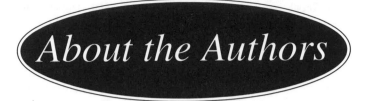
About the Authors

Dr. Semon and Ms. Kornblum are the authors of *Feast Without Yeast:4 Stages to Better Health* (1999), *An Extraordinary Power to Heal* (2003) and *Extraordinary Foods for the Everyday Kitchen* (2003). *Feast Without Yeast* has sold thousands of copies and is available throughout the world.

Dr. Bruce Semon is a board certified psychiatrist and child psychiatrist, as well as a doctorate level nutritionist, practicing in Milwaukee, Wisconsin. He received his M.D. from University of Wisconsin-Madison and his Ph.D. in Nutrition from University of California-Davis. Dr. Semon was a Research Fellow in the Laboratory of Nutritional and Molecular Regulation of the National Cancer Institute at the National Institutes of Health. He received his adult and child psychiatry training at the Medical College of Wisconsin.

Dr. Semon has published several academic papers relating to nutrition, and is a contributing author to *Biological Treatments for Autism and PDD*, by Dr. William Shaw.

As a complement to Dr. Semon's psychiatry practice, Dr. Semon has treated many patients for yeast-related illnesses with remarkable results. Dr. Semon speaks regularly to support groups and conferences about the connection between what people eat and their health.

Lori Kornblum is a graduate of Yale University and University of California-Boalt Hall Law School. She is an attorney practicing in Milwaukee, Wisconsin. She has published scholarly and popular articles relating to law. Ms. Kornblum has taught cooking classes to implement special diets and speaks about how to change diet.

Dr. Semon and Ms. Kornblum are married and live in Milwaukee with their three children, one of whom has an autistic disorder.

386

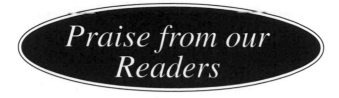

Praise from our Readers

"I just wanted to say that your book saved me. This cookbook is the best one I have found on the market. My children no longer feel deprived as they are on the road to better health." ---K.D.

"I have thoroughly enjoyed your book, *Feast Without Yeast.* I like yours better than some of the others because it's more practical and fits busy life-styles much better."   ---*Mary H.*

"Thank you so much for writing this book, and for the excellent recipes inside."   -----Ann H., Colorado

"As a parent of a child with a special need--Global Developmental delays--we've been searching for over 5 years for options that would help unlock the key to E's potential. This book has done more for us in the past 5 months since we've been following the diet than the last 5+ years of searching!" ----Ann. H., Wisconsin

"We are great admirers of your work and we have implemented many of your protocols for our son and my wife." ----Mike W.

"I wanted to thank you so much for your book."
                                                  ---Cherie

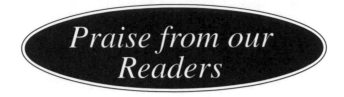

Praise from our Readers

"You will find a wealth of unbelievably tasty recipes in this well organized and easy to follow cookbook. Calling this a cookbook is a bit of an understatement, as you also get Dr. Semon's in-depth knowledge of nutrition, and the deeply touching narrative from Dr. Semon and Ms. Kornblum detailing their frustrating history of trying to treat their autistic son with any number of 'traditional' therapies, before discovering the benefits of a yeast-free diet. Highly recommended not only for the recipes, but for the wealth of nutritional information and the personal interest story."

----Jeff K., Portland

"I've read your excellent book, *Feast Without Yeast*, and I must say it is one of the best books of that type I have ever read. I think it will be a real treasure for many families in Yugoslavia. Your book means very much to me."

---Dr. Milijana Selakovic, Neuropsychiatrist, Belgrade

"We're on your recommended diet plus nystatin for about 10 weeks now. Y. changed dramatically in his willingness to eat foods that I never could dream he would eat---and that's so great!!!"

-----Abigail D., Israel